What's Up, Doc?

What's Up, Doc?

Dr Hilary Jones

BANTAM PRESS

LONDON · TORONTO · SYDNEY · AUCKLAND · JOHANNESBURG

TRANSWORLD PUBLISHERS
61–63 Uxbridge Road, London W5 5SA
A Random House Group Company
www.rbooks.co.uk

First published in Great Britain
in 2009 by Bantam Press
an imprint of Transworld Publishers

This book is a work of non-fiction based on the life, experiences and recollections of the
author. In some limited cases names of people, places, dates, sequences or the detail of
events have been changed to protect the privacy of others. The author has stated to the
publishers that, except in such minor respects, the contents of this book are true.

The information in this book is the professional opinion of Dr Hilary Jones but is not
a substitute and not to be relied on for medical, healthcare, pharmaceutical or other
professional advice on specific treatments in specific circumstances and in specific locations.
Please consult your GP before changing, stopping or starting any medical treatment. The
author and publishers disclaim, as far as the law allows, any liability arising directly or
indirectly from the use, or misuse, of the information contained in this book.

A CIP catalogue record for this book
is available from the British Library.

ISBN 9780593063712 (cased)
9780593063910 (tpb)

Addresses for Random House Group Ltd companies outside the UK
can be found at: www.randomhouse.co.uk
The Random House Group Ltd Reg. No. 954009

The Random House Group Limited supports The Forest Stewardship
Council (FSC), the leading international forest-certification organization. All our
titles that are printed on Greenpeace-approved FSC-certified paper carry the FSC logo.
Our paper procurement policy can be found at www.rbooks.co.uk/environment

Typeset in 12/15.5pt Sabon by
Falcon Oast Graphic Art Ltd

Printed and bound in Great Britain by
CPI Mackays, Chatham, ME5 8TD

2 4 6 8 10 9 7 5 3

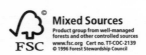

Mixed Sources
Product group from well-managed
forests and other controlled sources
www.fsc.org Cert no. TT-COC-2139
© 1996 Forest Stewardship Council
FSC

To Tris, Seb, Ru, Sammy and Dylan

CONTENTS

ACKNOWLEDGEMENTS

First and foremost I would like to thank all those hapless patients and friends of mine who have said they would be more than happy to share their intimate medical stories in this book with the rest of the world. So no issue of medical confidentiality there then. I think they all felt grateful to be helped out in a tight spot and are genuinely keen to have their problems written about on the basis that they may help other people and possibly give everyone a laugh at the same time. My thanks also to those wacky eccentrics out there who continually make medically orientated topics so interesting and controversial in the media, and all my medical colleagues who bail me out at the last minute with essential information just as I am due to go on air with breaking stories on rare and esoteric conditions.

I am indebted to David Miller, my brilliant literary agent, and to Doug Young, Rachel Walters and all the other lovely people at Transworld, to Prilly Brewin at Blue Stocking Limited, to Jo Spink PR, to Radio Lynx and to Colin Myler and Matt Nixson and others at the *News of the World* for being such great people to work with and write for.

I would like to give a special tribute to Peter McHugh, director of programmes at GMTV, for his enduring support, encouragement and loyalty, and to everyone else at GMTV with whom I have absolutely loved working, especially Martin Frizell, Michelle Porter, Emma Gormley, Ali Lutz, Anne Marie Leahy, Dave Mason, Mark Russell, Laura Hatton, Christina McDowall, Simon Jay, Trevor Le Jeune, Martin Petit, Jack Sandham, Beth Stratford and Nicki Johnceline. My fellow presenters have all been great – Penny Smith, Andrew Castle, Fiona Phillips and Lorraine Kelly especially. Sandra McKinney deserves a medal for putting up with her thankless task of being my PA at the Hampshire clinic. My thanks are also due to Steve Wright at Radio 2 for the gift of the 'skelington' and for bigging me up so frequently on his fantastic afternoon programme. Also to Dan Jones for the story about the pathology museum. I really hope your nose is now healed.

On a personal note, I would like to thank Dee Thresher for her endless love, trust, vitality and optimism, Kim and Bob Chapman for their boundless and unconditional support, and Yibi, whose pure beauty and generosity of spirit constantly remind me of the true value of life and humility long after he is no longer with us. I would like to thank Dr Bernie Graneek, without whose input I might well never have passed my final medical exams. Thanks, Bernie, for the answers to questions 4, 5 and 8 in that ridiculously irrelevant biochemistry practical.

Finally I would like to thank my parents, who always knew my career was destined to be in medicine and who showed me the importance of treating every person and patient as I would want to be treated myself. Thanks most of all, however, to all those people who have been on the receiving end of my medical attention and recipients of my personal brand of bedside manner. A medical degree is one thing but you taught me everything I really needed to know and continue to do so. May you live to a ripe old age in rude good health long after I hang up my stethoscope for the last time.

Introduction

To BE OR NOT TO BE? THAT IS NOT THE QUESTION. NOT FOR me anyway. For me the question is 'What's up, doc?' It has been ever since I qualified as a doctor at the Royal Free Hospital in London in 1976. When I was a junior medic, patients used to ask me, 'What's up, doc?' when I prodded their bellies for signs of appendicitis. On the GMTV sofa, presenters ask me, 'What's up with the latest actress who has developed the typical signs of anorexia nervosa?' In the tabloid newspapers, I'm asked to comment on what's up with the Premier League footballer who claims to suffer from sex addiction. On the radio I'm asked what's up with society in general, suffering as it does from epidemics of obesity and binge drinking.

But the question I'm being asked right now is of an altogether different nature. Not medical at all. I am at Elstree Studios on the set of *Celebrity Who Wants to Be a Millionaire?* and Chris Tarrant is asking me a question which, should I answer it correctly, will win a handsome £150,000 for charity. That's a lot of money. A huge amount of dosh to gamble away on an answer I am not really confident about. How many volunteers rattling their collection boxes on the high street on cold Saturday mornings would it take to make up for that kind of shortfall? Understandably, I'm feeling a tad nervous.

'What's up, doc?' enquires Chris ironically. 'A bad case of nerves? Palpitations? Tremor? Shall I ask the audience if there is a doctor in the house?' He is smiling gleefully, teasing out the tension and enjoying making me squirm.

Even the audience seems to be asking, 'What's up, doc? Why aren't you saying anything?'

But I'm used to answering questions, I tell myself. I probably answer hundreds of medical questions every week.

On an everyday basis in the GP surgery, people ask me about unexplained lumps in their neck, whether a pigmented mole is suspicious and should be removed or about the slurred speech and numbness in their face that they experienced the previous evening. Colleagues at work stop me in the corridor and ask about their child's leukaemia or their mum's dementia. People question me at dinner parties about their haemorrhoids, and in pubs on the merits of vasectomy. I've even been approached by complete strangers in dimly lit streets eager to hear my take on skunk and whether or not the NHS should freely supply methadone. And of course they ask me what Lorraine Kelly is really like.

At times I feel I may have made my medical opinion a little too accessible. You simply would not believe what intimate bodily secrets people impart to me when I'm down at the local enjoying a quiet pint. As one of the medical profession's better-known 'docs on the box', I suppose all this unsolicited attention is par for the course. To be fair, it is no more than I myself might inflict on some unsuspecting off-duty plumber, electrician or solicitor when I find myself stuck for a reliable opinion. Doctors learn very quickly never to let slip their title when introduced at social functions, and if they have any common sense at all they are reluctant to volunteer their services at sports arenas or in aircraft cabins at 30,000 feet when someone inconveniently collapses.

Although the programme is being recorded 'as live', the producers of *Celebrity Millionaire* have told me I can take as long as I like to respond to their questions and choose one of four possible options for my answer. So I do. I take an age. And in the meantime I cannot help but puzzle over how a bog-standard family GP with no major delusions of self-worth or grandeur ever got to be so widely recognized from TV and then ridiculously categorized as a 'celebrity' on a show like this. It has been an interesting story.

In June 1976 I officially became a proper doctor, a Bachelor of Medicine and a Bachelor of Surgery (MBBS), and was duly presented with an impressive-looking framed certificate to hang on the wall of my surgery if I felt I needed to prove it. The letters after my name were interpreted somewhat differently by my non-medical friends, who, having known me for years, insisted MBBS must stand for Medicine's Biggest Bullshitter. But despite their incredulity a doctor I most definitely now was, although I had to admit there had been many times when I'd needed to use considerable initiative to make it through the long six-year course. More of that later.

My medical career has been a fascinating journey. Among other places it's taken me to the island of Tristan da Cunha, a lonely volcanic outpost in the middle of the south Atlantic ocean and the most isolated inhabited island in the world. Here I worked single-handed as a medical officer and had to cope with everything nature and pathology could throw at me. There was no airstrip, it was outside helicopter range, well away from all regular shipping routes and the supply boat visited three times a year. From a medical perspective, apart from a few essential textbooks such as Harold Ellis's *Surgical Anatomy* and Geoffrey L. Howe's *The Extraction of Teeth*, I was, as they say, pretty much on my own. Not surprisingly, there were quite a few hairy moments. Once I had unpacked after a seven-day voyage on a 600-tonne fishing trawler, I immediately had to get to grips with the rather outdated anaesthetic machine, X-ray equipment and surgical instruments that had been left to gather cobwebs in the settlement's tiny hospital. When I look back I still think it's a miracle no one actually died on the island while I was in post. This was thanks partly to luck and partly to the excellent training I had had. I'd worked in casualty and ITU for a year at the hospital where I'd graduated before doing the usual medical and surgical stints for a further twelve months. There, working in a leukaemia and lymphoma unit then on an oncology ward and lastly with a general surgical team, I gained the variety of experience that junior doctors today might take three or four times longer to achieve. If we were on call, it was certainly not unusual to turn up at 8am on a Friday and work flat out until close of play at 8pm on Monday, if that was how long it took to make sure that the last patient's treatment had been completed satisfactorily. We did not get much sleep and it was common for us to be putting in one-hundred-hour weeks back to back. But we certainly learned how to detect an enlarged spleen or an abnormal liver, and to do something urgently about the first signs of septicaemia in a patient whose bone marrow had been cruelly displaced by aggressive cancer cells and who had no functional white cells with which to combat infection. It was a baptism of fire for sure. But it was an essential part of training and highly rewarding. It was also instrumental in giving me the confidence to do many of the things I subsequently chose to do, like working in Shetland for Offshore Medical Support and looking after the riggers, welders and laggers building the Sullom Voe oil refinery right up at the northernmost point of those inhospitable islands.

With TV-am I was given the opportunity to run in the New York marathon and stand in for Kathy Taylor as main presenter on her show when she was on maternity leave. At GMTV I was sent to snorkel off the Great Barrier Reef and saw my youngest child nearly fall out of the helicopter from which the camera crew had filmed. They had forgotten to replace the rear door for the return journey and eight-year-old Dylan very nearly went to swim with the sharks. I've been on trips to Lesotho to travel with the Philophepa Health Train as it provided basic care to the very poorest districts in that country. In the most moving interview I've ever done, I spoke to Yibi, at thirteen the oldest surviving child in South Africa who had been born with HIV. He talked so philosophically, without a trace of bitterness and with such mature calm, about the inevitable end of his own short but beautiful life. I released lions from wooden crates for the Born Free Organization at the Shamwari Game Reserve in South Africa and sedated white rhino with tranquillizing darts to tag them. I filmed 'healthy heart' strands in Buddhist temples in Japan. I carried out dental work on hyenas and performed surgery on pigs. So all in all it's been a wonderful journey of discovery. Time and time again my medical degree has proved the perfect ticket with which to travel the world and have a lot of fun while doing something constructive.

Ironically, it could all have been very different. I left

school with 'A' levels in English, History and French. Not ideal when you want to study medicine. However, I wasn't convinced at that time that a medical career was for me. I wasn't sure I could cope with all the boring physics and chemistry that I would be forced to cram in during a first-year conversion course in medicine. I had enjoyed a fantastic couple of years in the sixth form at Latymer Upper School in Hammersmith and, like so many of my schoolmates, I'd revelled in the theatrical activities of its Literary Guild. This club had done so much to nurture the acting careers of people like Mel Smith (I played Prince Hal to Mel's Falstaff in *Henry IV, Part One*), Chris and Dominic Guard, Alan Rickman and, several years later, Hugh Grant. But fun though it was, I couldn't identify a career in the arts that grabbed me. My dad's own antisocial hours as a busy GP were a bit of a turn-off and I realized that a junior doctor's pay was never going to allow me that Bose music centre or the Porsche. On the other hand, I'd always enjoyed the irreverence of *Doctor in the House* and the *Carry on Doctor* films and if becoming a doctor meant having a good laugh, drinking for England and dating nurses like the mini-skirted and buxom Barbara Windsor I reckoned it couldn't be all bad. Anyway, I figured it was only a six-year course – only! With a few more years of specialization at the end of it to look forward to, of course. Even if I hated it, I told myself, the qualification would be a lifelong passport opening doors in all branches of medicine all over the world. With a medical degree, careers beckoned in surgery, anaesthetics, general practice and pathology. Specializations in haematology, ophthalmology and interventional radiology offered fantastic prospects. But so did VSO work, clinical research and, ironically, I thought at the time, even medical journalism if I got desperate.

So perhaps it was destiny that nearly twenty years ago I wrote to the breakfast TV station TV-am and said, 'Gi's a job.' I felt the programme needed a more identifiable resident doc in the studio, someone the viewers could get to know and trust in much the same way that patients get to know and trust their own GP. I had already had fourteen years' experience in medical practice and I was keen to tell it like it is, willing to share a little bit of myself and my life with viewers. Most importantly, I was already relatively comfortable in front of TV cameras as I had been filming some of my patients for the last few years with a view to enhancing the education of trainee GPs. Much to my surprise, when they received my letter the bosses invited me up to the studios in Camden for an interview.

'You don't want your presenters to talk to all these different consultants every day as you have been doing,' I told them. 'These specialists are just people who know more and more about less and less until ultimately they know everything about nothing. They are boffins who confuse viewers with jargon, wear outdated bow ties and patronize. What you want is a media tart like me.'

By sheer coincidence, the charismatic if eccentric Australian MD of TV-am, Bruce Gyngell, had actually been looking for a regular doctor to cover most of the medical issues on a daily basis and he agreed. They offered me a fortnight's trial on the sofa talking about subjects as mundane as high blood pressure and varicose veins, and fortunately the response from viewers was good. A long-term contract was duly offered and I signed it without a thought for my GP colleagues, who I suspected might be rather miffed. That was an underestimate. But at least I was happy.

This was what I really wanted to do. I'd been incredibly busy for nearly ten years in NHS general practice, looking after 2,700 patients on my personal list, and I needed a fresh challenge. I could easily juggle the two jobs and besides, I argued to myself, the roles would be complementary. My patients would tell me what people most needed to hear on TV about medical issues, and the research I carried out prior to the programmes would benefit my patients as I would undoubtedly become more up to date with the latest treatments. All I had to do was get used to very little sleep.

For over a year I worked full-time in general practice, spending every fifth night and weekend on call as well. Then, in 1990, despite significant sleep deprivation, I managed to run the New York marathon for TV-am in my holiday time. I vaguely remember doing a live interview with Lorraine Kelly from a tiny studio in Times Square fourteen hours after the event, feeling extremely tired and very, very drunk. No one seemed to notice. Everyone interpreted the hyper-excitable non-stop gabbling as euphoria and relief.

Bruce then came up with the brilliant idea of positioning the 'doc spot', as he called it, adjacent to the entertainment slot. This regular feature was generally regarded as the most watched part of the programme. So within a few weeks this ordinary common-or-garden family doctor found himself sitting next to the likes of Dudley Moore, Charlton Heston, Lennox Lewis and Joan Rivers and chatting about everything medical they cared to bring up. It was intense, enjoyable, informative and fun. In fact it was mainly the informal banter that made the doc spot so popular. People learned about medicine while having a good laugh. Dudley Moore even managed to laugh when my six-month-old son Ru threw up all over his best suit on live TV. It was 'infotainment' at its best, and judging by the ratings it seemed to work.

Next, not long after I joined TV-am, the *News of the World* offered me my own column answering readers' health questions and speculating on the medical afflictions of the glitterati. As a media medic, I've now been publicly commenting on the physical and psychological health of celebrities for more than twenty years. You could say I've been 'seeing stars' for a very long time.

Whether it's on TV, radio or in tabloid newspapers and glossy magazines, not a single day passes without banner headlines devoted to either the medical misfortune or the remarkable rehabilitation of someone rich and famous. Sometimes a source of amusement, and sometimes of shock, scepticism or sadness, the medical trials and tribulations of TV personalities, singers, sportsmen, models and politicians fascinate us because we cannot help but be intrigued by how they cope with the very same symptoms and ailments that can touch each and every one of us. Also, because they tend to be so frank about their problems, warts and all, they can often highlight medical issues and educate the public more effectively than us doctors. Whether it's John Prescott's bulimia, Kylie Minogue's breast cancer, Naomi Campbell's air rage, Max Mosley's non-Nazi-themed bondage sessions or Kerry Katona's drug-fuelled pregnancy, we are all desperate to identify, at least to some extent, with these most humanizing experiences of the superstars.

Combined with the everyday but often bizarre world of routine general practice and the constant developments in medical research that come my way, my media career has been a privilege and an essential part of what the General Medical Council would call my 'continuing medical education'. It's not been without a few good laughs either – many of which have been entirely at my own expense.

I

All in a Day's Work

FRANK BRUNO WAS ON THE GMTV SOFA ONE DAY TALKING about his recovery from severe depression. We were doing a whole week's strand on the subject and had already had a phenomenal response to our interviews about post-natal and childhood depression. Our hope was that Frank, as a high-profile and popular personality, would help raise awareness of the symptoms and dispel much of the un-deserved social stigma that accompanies the condition, and we weren't disappointed.

I'd met Frank a few times over the years and I'd always found him humble, very approachable and great fun. So did the British public, obviously, as all the guests in the crowded Green Room stood and made a fuss of him. Frank is one of those major celebrities who have attained 'national treasure' status in all our hearts and minds, not just because he was a fantastic athlete and boxer but also because he came from a lowly background, proved himself the hard way, and then fell spectacularly from grace as a result of domestic issues and mental illness.

In 1995 Frank had beaten Oliver McCall at Wembley Stadium to become WBC World Heavyweight Champion. He was at the peak of his career, having finally achieved his elusive and overarching ambition and then celebrated by buying the very boxing ring in which he'd done it. We undoubtedly loved him just for that, but to a much greater degree we loved him for his gentle giant demeanour, his humility and his unmistakable deep, rumbling belly laugh. His knockabout repartee with BBC commentator Harry Carpenter, usually signed off with his trademark 'Ya know what I mean, Harry', was legendary. But by 2003, a messy divorce, the end of his boxing career and the tragic apparent suicide of his former trainer, George Francis, had all contributed to the gradual onset of increasingly bizarre and illogical behaviour that was finally diagnosed at Goodmayes Hospital in Ilford as depression and bipolar disorder.

Front-page headlines on the day he was sectioned under the Mental Health Act were predictably insensitive. The *Sun* ran with 'BONKERS BRUNO LOCKED UP' at first, only to change it to 'SAD BRUNO IN MENTAL HOME' when they thought better of it. The chief executive of the charity SANE was moved to say at the time, 'It is both an insult to Mr Bruno and damaging to the many thousands of people who endure mental illness to label him "bonkers" or "a nutter" and having to be "put in a mental home".' We at GMTV couldn't have agreed more and that was why we now had him on our sofa looking like a million dollars and resplendent in a perfectly tailored suit and tie, with bespoke blue-leather shoes on his outsized feet.

Frank and I entered the studio for the 6am news hour, and John Stapleton welcomed him warmly and gently enquired about what he could remember of the days leading up to his admission to hospital. 'It was a very low time for me,' he said. 'I didn't know whether I was depressed or not – everything was a blur.' Then he described how much he missed the day-to-day life he'd had in boxing, the discipline of the training, the physicality of the fights and the buzz and excitement of press conferences and everything that went with them. I couldn't help thinking that this sudden loss of everything that he stood for, and the gradual slide down from the giddy heights of international stardom to mediocrity and ordinariness, must be a harrowing period in the life of anyone who has ever experienced the thrill of fame and public adoration. How many hundreds of one-time superstars have been damaged or even destroyed by their own inability to make the necessary adjustments in their personal lives to blend in to normal existence?

The loss of his wife Laura, through divorce, his trainer through death and his boxing career through age must have hit him like a sledgehammer. Three bereavements all in a row. And some of us are simply much better able to cope than others. John then asked Frank how he was coping now. 'Back to much happier times by the look of you?' John added. 'Yeah, yeah, oh definitely – still ducking and diving, heh, heh, heh, you know what I mean. Obviously I'm not with Laura so I can get a bit lonely.' John paused momentarily, only to hear Frank continue with the immortal words, 'But you get to know what your right and left hands are for, if you know what I mean, heh, heh, heh.' John and I looked at each other. Had Frank just alluded to what we thought he was alluding to? Yes, he had. And to my knowledge, it was the first time in eighteen years on the GMTV sofa that any reference had ever been made to masturbation. In the news hour anyway. So we moved swiftly on and nobody else bar the grinning cameraman seemed to bat an eyelid.

Later, in the 7am main programme, it was Fiona Phillips's turn to chat to Frank, who was now perfectly warmed up for his finale. Asking about his treatment, she said, 'You even had to have injections in your backside, didn't you?' To which Frank replied, 'Well, not right in my backside, no. They were just to the right or left of it, heh, heh, heh.' It was silly but completely hilarious and only boosted Frank's popularity the more.

An hour later as I drove back down the M3 to my surgery in Hampshire I couldn't help thinking what a constructive and entertaining chap Frank had been. He had managed in an interview of less than four minutes to do more to abolish the stigma of mental illness and to promote the message that yes, you can make a full recovery from it, than any number of media doctors or mental health care charities could have achieved in a week. The avalanche of calls recorded in our duty telephone log had accurately reflected that fact, with many members of the public also bidding Frank the very best of luck and good health in the future.

Frank was once again a true champion that day, only this time fighting for those who've suffered from depression and proving that it's perfectly OK to stand up and admit you've been depressed, fought the battle and won the fight even after a serious knockdown. For that at least, he'll always be one of my heroes.

Later on in the afternoon reality caught up with me and I came back down to earth with a bump. I was in my GP clinic and there was a patient sitting in front of me with half his ear missing. And it wasn't a pretty sight. It looked like the top two inches had been gnawed off by a giant rat. One of the extraordinary things about medicine is that every-body's attitude towards health and disease is different. At one end of the spectrum there are people who will rush to see the doctor for the least little thing. A twinge here, an ache there, a tiny lump or bump or a minor nasal sniffle of ten minutes' duration. At the other end are the people who are so stoic they would rather eat their own eyeballs than waste the good doctor's time for something as trivial as bronchial pneumonia, a strangulated hernia or even a mild heart attack. With only 75 per cent of his full complement of ears, Simon James was firmly in the latter camp.

It is difficult to know exactly why some people are so reluctant to visit the doctor when clearly something is terribly wrong. Very often they dread having their worst fears confirmed. They are also terrified, sometimes, of the imagined indignities of treatment. Embarrassment is a factor if the problem is below the waist, but discomfort too, at having to expose themselves to the invasive examinations, judgemental comments and perceived arrogance of uncaring doctors. Maybe that was why Dorothy's breast cancer had taken so long to be discovered. She had eventually come to see me about a 'skin rash'. It turned out that her cancer was so advanced that the tumour had eroded through the skin and was completely exposed on the surface of the areola surrounding the nipple.

It probably explains why Douglas told nobody about his impressive scrotal hydrocele until he could no longer find a pair of trousers he could squeeze into. The surgeons aspirated 1.5 litres of fluid from the sac around his testicle before he was restored to normal. Now I'm pleased to say he comes to see me more regularly and with less reluctance. In size-32-waist slim-fit trousers.

Thankfully, such isolated instances of extreme self-neglect are much less common than they used to be. Nevertheless there in front of me was Simon James, a fifty-two-year-old agricultural worker whose medical records told me he hadn't seen a doctor for twenty-seven years. Not since he had had a tetanus booster following an accident with a pitchfork. His whole demeanour suggested a loathing of visits to the doctor and I was sure he had come in this time only on sufferance.

'I think I've got an infection on my ear,' he said.

'How long do you think it's been going on?' I asked.

''Bout a month or two. Maybe a bit longer.'

'Let's take a closer look.'

I already knew exactly what the problem was. Yes, there was infection. But the bacterial infection causing the redness and weeping was secondary to the underlying condition, which was a severely neglected basal cell carcinoma. These skin cancers are the commonest and most benign of all skin cancers and classically appear in exposed areas such as the facial triangle between the eye, mouth and ear.

'Simon, you don't really like doctors, do you?'

'Well, no, not really.'

'And that's why you don't come to see them very often. To tell you the truth, I don't have much time for them either. Arrogant gits, most of them. But I'll be totally straight with you. I want to help you get this cleared up. How long have you really had it, by the way?'

'Couple of years. Just sort of grew slowly. Never bothered me much.'

'It wouldn't. You work on a farm. You're not an Armani model, are you? There's not a vain cell in your body. But the ear does need treatment. What you've got there is a rodent ulcer. It's a benign type of skin cancer which starts off as a tiny spot like an insect bite. You get a small ulcer crater which scabs over and then the scab falls off and builds up again as the ulcer slowly enlarges. But this kind of cancer never spreads anywhere else. It can't kill you like other cancers. What this cancer does do, however, is gradually eat away at the surrounding tissue just like a rat chews on a piece of gristle. That's why it's called a rodent ulcer.'

The most severe example I'd ever seen was in a pathology specimen jar at the Wellcome Museum in London during my student days. Inside the jar, bathed in formalin, was the head of a nineteenth-century sailor whose untreated rodent ulcer had eaten the front of his face away. The eye socket was empty, half the nose gone, the nerves and blood vessels exposed for all to see. How the poor man had lived so long without succumbing to death from septicaemia was simply incredible. It was an image that was difficult to forget.

At least Simon could have curative treatment before his rodent ulcer progressed further. I explained that his treatment would consist of surgery to remove the remaining cancer, although radiology was an alternative. Because much of the cartilage had been destroyed, reconstructive surgery to repair the ear would also be available should he want it. He calmly accepted what I said as if he had suspected something like this all along, and agreed for me to refer him for urgent assessment. I was glad that he seemed to feel he could talk to me as he promised to call me if he thought of any questions. Whether or not he would actually turn up for his hospital appointment, though, was anyone's guess. I certainly hoped he would.

Two hours later that same evening and I was back at home, with Bill the plumber working on a new en-suite shower room for Sammy, my teenage daughter. He asked me if I could possibly get him a signed photograph of Penny Smith, the presenter of *Newshour* on GMTV. Apparently he quite fancied her. Well, there's no accounting for taste, is there?

17

Plumbers aren't exactly renowned for their appreciation of elegance and beauty after all. But since I wanted the shower room finished to everyone's satisfaction I duly promised to acquire the photo. Now Penny is a bit of a pushover when it comes to this sort of thing because she loves the idea of a bloke having the hots for her and she likes nothing more than scribbling an outrageous bit of innuendo on her publicity photographs. We all share a joke in the mornings in the TV studio and take the mickey out of each other mercilessly. The central character in her first novel, *Coming Up Next*, is not at all unlike her.

'Penny,' I asked her the following morning, 'can you do a signed photo for my plumber, Bill, who obviously likes butch women? Can you write a suitably rude message on it as well?'

'Sure,' said Penny, 'leave it with me.'

One week later she asked how the personalized gift had gone down.

'But you haven't given it to me yet,' I replied.

'Yes I have, I signed it, wrote a suggestive message on it and popped it into your briefcase in the Green Room.'

'What briefcase?'

'The brown one.'

'I don't have a brown briefcase . . .'

'Who the hell was in the Green Room that day last week then?' she asked in something of a panic.

She had turned a little pale at this point and I couldn't help smirking as I asked what her message had said.

'It said,' she muttered thoughtfully, '"The next time I want my pipes rodded I shall now know where to come."'

I burst out laughing as we both frantically looked at the previous week's running order to see who the lucky recipient of the message could possibly have been. And there it was. We

18

had had only one guest that day. Penny had unwittingly delivered her message to . . . the ambassador for Saudi Arabia.

Seven days later, Penny was still wondering what the high-ranking officials at the Saudi Arabian Embassy could possibly be saying about her and her raunchy signed photograph.

'It's not exactly brilliant for my reputation, is it?' she said.

'No,' I replied. 'Especially as it's been a whole week and the ambassador hasn't even been in touch yet.'

Around us producers, guests, greeters and runners were sniggering. Yet another typical day in the office at GMTV.

The real purpose of my presence in front of the cameras that day, however, was to comment on a bearded man who was having a baby and who was defying the sceptics who said it was just an April fool's joke. Just like the one GMTV had played for real in much the same vein several years previously. But transgender man Thomas Beatie was far from being an April fool's joke. He was definitely born a woman and had decided to become a man ten years previously by having his breasts surgically removed and taking the male hormone testosterone. Chromosomally, biologically and anatomically he was a woman, but legally in the US where he lived he was a man. So I couldn't help thinking that I had to get the terminology right on this one or I would end by upsetting everyone – transgenders, trans-sexuals, gays, lesbians, heterosexuals, the lot. This subject was about as PC as it could possibly get.

Because Thomas hadn't had his reproductive organs removed and had discontinued his testosterone medication, there was no physiological reason why he couldn't conceive and give birth to a baby. He and his female partner had bought sperm from a sperm bank and inseminated him using a turkey baster. With his wispy little goatee beard and all. Confused? We all were. As I suspected the child might be when he or she was finally delivered and grew up to realize his or her parents weren't quite like other parents.

But it's always easy to sit in judgement and on TV it's crucial for any medical professional to be impartial and objective. This couple would certainly have their detractors and there would be millions of people willing to condemn them. But were they really any different from a lesbian or gay couple legally adopting a baby? And wasn't their ability to nurture a child greater than that of any heterosexual couple who neglected or abused their own baby but weren't questioned by society in any way? Transgenderism is an area that even the most liberal-minded of people still have problems getting their head around.

Predictably, perhaps, Thomas Beatie was not going to stay out of the news for long. A few weeks later I was down in the South of France filming a strand called 'Beach Surgery' for breakfast TV when I got a call from Matt, my ex-page editor from the *News of the World*. He was horrified to hear that I was in a gay.

'No,' I said carefully, 'Agay. It's a nice little place on the sea near St Raphael. What's up?'

Apparently transgender man was in the news again because the baby that he gave birth to was being breastfed by his wife. Could I comment? Was it remotely possible that a woman who hadn't recently had a baby or been pregnant could successfully breastfeed? If so, how could that happen?

In days gone by, well-to-do mothers used to hand over their newborn babies for wet nursing. This meant that a surrogate lactating mother would put the baby to her own breast in order to feed it and spare the real mother the pleasure. But wet nurses would already be lactating as a result of a previous pregnancy. They would not have allowed their milk to dry up, either by breastfeeding continuously or by constantly expressing their milk. But this particular woman had not been pregnant or lactating for years. Could she possibly have stimulated her own breasts and nipples sufficiently to successfully nourish her baby? Almost certainly not. There have been anecdotal instances of this happening but evidence is scarce and scientifically it makes no sense. You need the hormones prolactin and oxytocin to generate milk production. You need the milk ducts to be primed by high levels of circulating oestrogen for many months in order for this to occur. So could she have taken artificial hormones prescribed by her doctor, just as her husband did when he took testosterone to change from a woman into a man? Possibly, but I had never heard of such a case.

So what was my view? The mother was putting this baby to the breast solely for psychological 'bonding' purposes, I thought. All nutritional succour was coming from formula milk given by bottle. Transgender man, who delivered the baby, hadn't got any breast tissue as he'd had it surgically removed when he had his partial sex change. The couple had always said they wanted to raise the baby together, equally, and with love, and presumably they were simply doing their best to share out the family duties.

Wet nursing these days is ill-advised. The risk of transmitting hepatitis and HIV among other things makes it potentially hazardous. There are safer and more appropriate alternatives, although the La Leche League and the Association for Breastfeeding Mothers would almost certainly take issue with me – they often do. But at the end of the day, this baby was not being breastfed in the traditional sense – but then this baby's future was not going to be a conventional one anyway.

Matt was grateful for my comments and said so.

'Has the baby been named yet, by any chance?' I asked. 'I hope to God it's not Hilary.'

People often tell me – well, other doctors who aren't on telly do – what a fantastic perk it must be to swan off to beautiful places like St Raphael and be put up in five-star hotels at someone else's expense. Yes, but it is hard work – especially in the full glare of the Mediterranean sun while being constantly tempted by the culinary delights of the local seafood and fine white wines. Once I even had to ask the waiter for another egg on my Caesar salad. After all, as Giscard d'Estaing once said, 'One egg on its own is some- times not an oeuf.' Yes, a trip like this took its toll but hey, someone had to do it.

If transgender man Thomas Beatie's story was not bizarre enough, the TV appearance of Ellen Greve was even more peculiar. Occasionally, TV companies like to invite someone really wacky on to the show knowing that their opinions will incite amazement, excitement, disbelief or anger. They know that whatever they have to say will be so far removed from what most people consider to be normal that it is bound to create a reaction. And good TV ratings as a result. My interview with Ellen Greve was a prime example. This not unattractive and gentle-sounding Australian lady pro- fessed to be a Breatharian. She belonged to a cult that proclaims that people can live on fresh air alone. The cult's activities had already engendered a fair amount of media coverage, and three deaths in Scotland had been attributed to the victims' obsessively following its techniques. An investigative journalist had also apparently caught the cult's leader red-handed, emerging from a burger bar somewhere north of the border. Now we had Ellen Greve in our studio in Edinburgh talking to me 'down the line' on the GMTV sofa in London. I was relishing the chance to chat directly with her, and straight after she had spouted on ridiculously for a minute or two of complete spiritual psycho-babble the lovely Kate Garraway kicked off with a question for me.

'Hilary,' she said, 'less than three hundred calories a day and getting your nourishment from an outside source? What do you make of that?'

'Well, it's nonsense,' I replied. 'I simply don't believe a word of it, and I don't know whether this lady knows how dangerous she is and how insulting she's being to the third world by suggesting that people can live off divine light.'

Ellen Greve came back at me. 'When you've found a solution for world health and hunger-related problems like we have,' she said, 'which is in my book *Ambassadors of Light*, now available in Britain, there is data of how we can save these children who are dying at a rate of one every second, so I've yet to meet a doctor who's spent any time studying Prana or even knows what Prana is. I've yet to meet a doctor who has seen the power of the divine force—'

'It's interesting you're waving your book,' I said to her, interrupting her nonsense in full flow. 'I hope that no one buys it. I think it's drivel, I think it's dangerous, I think you are deluded, I don't think you have any evidence at all to back up what you are saying and we have had three deaths associated with your cult, and we've also had an Australian television programme called *60 Minutes* expose you as a fraud – I really don't know why you're getting air time. You are a self-publicist and I think you are dangerous.'

In my earpiece, the producers and director in the gallery were whooping with glee at my unexpected rant, knowing full well that I rarely laid into people with venom and that, whatever the outcome, it was making great telly. You always knew when it had because later in the day you got ten times as many comments by phone, fax and text as you usually did, with most of your mates ripping into you and saying what a cruel bastard you had been. I have to say I had meant every word of it.

As I made my way back upstairs from the studio to the newsroom, it was clear that all the overnight staff who had been watching the item had thoroughly enjoyed it. 'Way to go, doc,' said one as he lolled in front of his computer. 'About time to come off the fence! Why didn't you tell her what you *really* felt?'

Smiling, with a curious feeling of satisfaction, I picked up one of the day's well-thumbed newspapers. The tragic knife murder of yet another teenager was all over it. A knife can kill a human being in a single apparently effortless thrust. Ask any forensic pathologist. We have so many of them on the box these days. *Dangerfield. Silent Witness. Waking the Dead.* A knife pushed vertically between the ribs just hits bone and comes to an abrupt halt. It hurts like hell but seldom causes much lasting damage. But the same blade thrust horizontally slices easily through skin, adipose tissue and intercostal muscle before entering the chest cavity, where nothing really impedes its path until it bursts the lung and ruptures the heart muscle. Torrential bleeding, enhanced by the heart's pumping action, quickly fills the pericardium, its membranous covering, constricting the heart itself in a fatal embrace called cardiac tamponade. The few moments it takes for this to happen enable the victim to stagger those few last yards before gasping for help or making a last desperate phone call. The end thereafter is swift. They have 'bled out' – lost ten or more litres of vital oxygen-carrying blood from their abdomen, chest cavity or neck.

Something similarly random occurs with intracranial bleeding. A steel toecap to the side of the head can deliver enormous pressure per square inch of skull. Usually the bone is simply pushed inwards and becomes physically depressed. But occasionally, at a critical location one inch in front of and one inch above the ear, the splintering bone fragments will sever an artery and cause a classic subdural haemorrhage. Subdurals are the most feared injuries of professional boxers, who may or may not be knocked unconscious during the bout but who subsequently collapse and have to undergo urgent neurosurgery to save their life. I was once deeply involved in such a drama when, as a junior doctor, I was called to see a man who had been dealt a glancing blow on the side of the head by a bus as it pulled into the bus stop where he had been waiting. An hour later, fully compos mentis, he walked into A&E with nothing more than a mild headache but quickly slipped into a coma in the few minutes it took for me to examine him. The pupil of one eye was fully dilated compared to the other, smaller one and stubbornly refused to react to light as it should have done. His pulse was abnormally slow and his blood pressure alarmingly high. The diagnosis of subdural haemorrhage was clear. Without hesitation I bleeped the excellent senior registrar, Mr Charlie Weston (not his real name), who I knew to be supping a well-deserved pint across the road from the Royal Free Hospital after a long day's cutting in the operating theatre. Within a moment he was there.

'Sister,' he yelled through the cubicle curtains after taking a quick look, 'fetch me a burrhole set now.' A burrhole is a circular hole drilled through the skull with the express aim of releasing the blood trapped beneath the bone that is causing pressure on the brain and constriction of the vital structures within it. It's a centuries-old procedure called

25

trephining and many an ancient skull discovered by archae-
ologists bears evidence of human interference carried out in
the name of surgery, tribal ritual or plain superstition. 'You
can't open his skull here,' protested the senior nurse. 'We'll
have to prepare theatre.'

'No time, we'll lose him.'

But we didn't. Without anaesthetic, Charlie expertly
drilled a burrhole and as fresh red blood squirted out on to
the pillow our patient began to come round. The anaes-
thetist summoned earlier and arriving at that instant quickly
sedated the patient so that we could carry on and stabilize
his condition. It was one of the most dramatic surgical
experiences I have ever had and Charlie, by flying in the face
of accepted protocol and not waiting to take the patient to
theatre, undoubtedly saved this man's life. There would not
have been enough time otherwise. What we did would
rarely happen today, and if it did it would probably result in
some politically correct disciplinary action. But the patient
made a full recovery and was able to walk out of the
hospital when he was discharged five days later. He was one
of the lucky ones.

Many patients with subdural haemorrhages and knife
wounds, from whatever cause, simply do not make it. It is
random and it is unpredictable and this is especially true of
deliberate stabbings. Alarmingly, tabloid headlines showed
that more than fifty people were killed by stabbing in
London alone in 2008. My colleagues working in casualty
departments could hardly keep up with the carnage.

This frightening increase in teenage knife attacks has pan-
icked the nation and prompted the suggestion that the
perpetrators and those who carry knives should visit A&E
departments to see for themselves the appalling injuries
suffered by stab victims. The idea, I suppose, is that feral

youths from criminal gangs who believe only in physical dominance and aggression to succeed in life will suddenly develop a conscience and miraculously mend their ways when confronted by a traumatized victim with a nice clean medicated dressing taped to their skin. As an ex-casualty officer I cannot believe the naivety of such a suggestion. Guys who carry knives rarely have a conscience. They do not care much about being part of civilized society and generally see showing remorse as a fatal weakness. The Royal College of Surgeons seems to agree on this. They described the plan as 'distasteful' and 'morally, ethically and legally suspect'. But I'm sure it is the case that few of these thugs actually set out deliberately to kill their victims. After all, people who spare no thought for the welfare of their victims might think twice about an action that could well result in a very inconvenient stretch inside one of Her Majesty's prisons and an embarrassing loss of face among their peer group.

People are being murdered simply because the thugs concerned have no idea how frail the human body really is. The violence used is often frenetic and prolonged, yet the dividing line between delivering a damned good beating and actually causing death can easily be overstepped. A metal blade of any length may sever a major artery or penetrate the heart. But I do not believe the murderers' aim or knowledge of anatomy is in reality that good. These people watch cartoon characters on television, see them getting squashed flat or blown up and genuinely think the human body can recover from similar injuries with equal impunity. Sometimes, almost miraculously, it can – but just as the events leading up to the assault are random, so an attack using a knife can unhappily result in death. This is the lottery of premeditated violence fuelled by warped ideas based on a gang culture of 'respect', a morbid fear of losing face and intoxication from alcohol and other drugs.

Unfortunately the statistics warn of worse to come. Perhaps the beginning of a breakdown in the basic fabric of society. Almost 14,000 people every year are victims of knife attacks in the UK, with convictions for carrying a knife doubling in the decade from 1997 to 6,314 in 2006. Yet for every attack reported or conviction registered for carrying, you can multiply these figures significantly. In 2008 there was a 75 per cent rise over the last five years in teenagers being admitted to hospital with serious stab wounds. But will the government's £100 million youth crime action plan be enough to stem this crimson tide of death by haemorrhage?

The head of a new anti-knife-crime team, Mr Hitchcock (ironically named as Alfred Hitchcock's famous film *Psycho* centred on a frenzied knife attack in the shower), plans a non-military version of national service. Jacqui Smith, Home Secretary at the time of writing, plans to introduce knifers to their victims. Curfews are suggested to clear the streets of under-sixteens after 9pm in knife crime hotspots. But will it be enough to make a real difference? The government can pussyfoot all they like with half-baked gimmicks such as national service, community service and attempts to appeal to the underlying decency of violent criminals by arranging cosy meetings with their traumatized victims. But prison works, provided it is a genuine deterrent, and perhaps this is where any social rehabilitation should take place. Not at the expense of disabled or elderly people, who would probably be horrified if they realized they were being palmed off with such dubious helpers as has been suggested.

Just serving time may not be enough, though. Having

to forgo some of the freedoms that society bestows on individuals, such as the right to drive a car, might help. Certainly right now the incentives for young men to give up their weapons and their violent way of life are too few. Among other things, we need more imaginative and charismatic leaders at every level to show the disaffected and feral youth of today that there can be another way. We have to hope so because some people (especially those who have lost loved ones to knife crime) might otherwise say that the only practical alternative is selective youthanasia.

Just as all this morbid rumination about death and dying was beginning to depress me, Penny Smith breezed into the newsroom and cheered me up. She always claims she has been forty-three for at least five years so I couldn't resist telling her about an article I'd just read saying that human ageing was about to be solved through the study of the genes of fruit flies. Without missing a beat, she fired a suitable riposte straight back.

'Time flies like an arrow,' she said. 'Fruit flies like a banana.'

She is mad. Where does she get this stuff from? One other independent doctor's signature on a special form together with mine and I could easily have her sectioned under the Mental Health Act. I have to say the prospect is quite tempting.

2

WHAT'S IN A NAME?

I WAS JOINING STEVE WRIGHT ON HIS RADIO 2 SHOW ONE DAY, as I do every six weeks or so, and the lovely Tim Smith and Janey Lee Grace were there as well. I love doing Steve's show because we chat about topical medical subjects and manage to have a bit of a giggle while addressing the serious issues as well. I started by telling him that a doctor from Cambridge University had published an article where she argued that old-fashioned medical jargon based on Greek and Latin derivations of words 2,000 years old are confusing patients and putting their lives at risk.

Hyper, meaning too much, and hypo, meaning too little, can easily be confused in written text or in conversation, yet treatment for hyperglycaemia is the total opposite to the treatment for hypoglycaemia. Inter means between, and intra means within, so a senior doctor giving instructions to a junior and shouting them across a busy casualty department might end up with the patient having an injection in the wrong place. But it turned out that Steve, Tim and Janey quite liked medical jargon and didn't want it dumbed down.

They liked the fact that doctors describe the common cold as an upper respiratory tract infection, and post-viral fatigue as myalgic encephalomyelitis. They enjoyed the mystique of halux vulgus as opposed to the domesticity of the word bunion, while I pointed out that the words sub-acute sclerosing panencephalitis perfectly describe a condition that would otherwise require a whole paragraph of explanation.

I also mentioned that doctors sometimes deliberately use jargon so that the patient doesn't understand. If I said that Tim had a supratentorial lesion and wrote it in his medical notes, I'd be saying that all his problems were in his mind. If I said he was neuronally challenged, I'd be saying the same thing. Janey and Tim looked bemused. Steve simply added, 'And I think you'd be right.'

After the show, somebody asked me a question I must have been asked millions of times over the years – but much more so recently since I became a doctor on the telly.

How does any self-respecting bloke get to be called Hilary? I mean *Hilary*, isn't that a girl's name? What was it like being mercilessly teased at school by groups of mocking youths who reckoned I must at best be a bit of a sissy or at worst a complete poof? And no, it wasn't a mix-up in the maternity ward as a result of ambiguous genitalia. There are photos to prove it. My name actually came about because, the day before I was born, Edmund Hillary had done what no other man had ever done before in the history of the world. He had conquered Everest. Such was my parents' elation and admiration for this landmark achievement that I suspect my name was always going to be Hilary whichever sex I turned out to be. But for some bizarre reason, only one 'l' and not two.

'A great and noble explanation, Dad,' I'd say ten years

later, on returning from school with yet another bloody nose and split lip from fighting my corner after being called a girlie. 'But why couldn't I have had a bog-standard name like my brothers Nick, David and Huw – even Edmund for that matter? It would have been a lot easier. As it is, every day it's like the Johnny Cash song "A Boy Named Sue". Only it's worse. It's Hilary.' But my protests fell on deaf ears. Such was my dad's passion for pioneering in general and mountaineering in particular, he just didn't get it. He couldn't see the problem. 'We could have called you Tenzing Norgay, I suppose,' he once conceded. 'But we may never discover who actually stepped on the summit first.' A sympathetic sort of bloke, my dad.

Later, the name proved instrumental in getting me into medical school. When I applied for a place to study medicine, I'd accompanied my UCCA form with a letter signed Hilary Jones. At the interview it was clear the previous four students had had a tough time in front of the panel of academics and professors, who had obviously given them a grilling. But when I walked in they all fell about laughing, having expected to see a woman called Hilary as their medical school had traditionally been a women-only teaching hospital. We talked about little else for the full twenty minutes of the interview, so all in all it was a bit of a doddle. The name had got me in.

In time the name became even less of a handicap and when the TV career finally began it turned out, much to my surprise, to be something of a bonus. With a common surname like Jones, Hilary sort of stood out. Dr Hilary had a certain cachet and curiosity value, whereas Dr Dave, Bob or Fred possibly might not have done. Especially as the doctor concerned was pretty obviously a bloke. Well, I like to think so anyway.

Ever since I finally came to terms with my nominal inheritance I have had a certain fascination for names. Like the NHS patient whose surname was Koch and whose Christian name was Everard. I would not have believed it, had I not seen his medical notes with my own eyes. I once knew someone called Holdon who as a boy would wet himself on a daily basis. Is it really possible that the name given to us can actually influence our future career and behaviour? Am I the only person who reads newspaper stories and is struck by the aptness of the name of the central character? The burglar called Nick, the archaeologist called Robin Graves, the decorator called Painter, the stunt man called Reckless or the stalker with one eye and a lisp called Strange? In Hammersmith I used to pass an optician called Seymour on my way home from school. A few yards further down the road was a dentist called Phang. Do you see where I'm coming from here? To me the coincidences seem far too frequent for the link between the name and the career to be happening by chance. Could there really be a nominal destiny that shapes our ends? It was a puzzle and I needed to work it out.

I decided to carry out a small scientific experiment. I consulted a huge tome called *The Official UK Medical Directory* that listed every registered doctor in the country and their speciality. And bingo! I quickly found a disproportionate number of orthopaedic surgeons called Bone, haematologists called Blood, sex counsellors called Love and neurologists called Brain. I even found a skin specialist called Cream, a urologist running an erectile dysfunction clinic called Horne and a forensic pathologist named De'Ath. Spooky, eh? The name Hilary, for all its early unwelcome consequences, was at least career-neutral as far as medical specialization was concerned. It was often shortened to Hil by people too embarrassed to come out with all three girlie syllables, or to Hils, or sometimes, particularly in the East End, to just plain 'H'. At least it was different. So to all the Lindsays, Leslies, Robins, Valeries, Kims and Francises whose names are also gender-ambiguous, I say just remember how much tougher you have to become to conquer the hurdle. What doesn't kill us will only make us stronger. What's in a name anyway?

When you think about it, the most important thing to do is to get the name right when you initially meet someone. In the past, my father had found this out the hard way. It was years before the advent of computerized screens in waiting rooms and at a time when doctors were still sometimes thought of as gods. Patients never questioned anything. My dad, like all the other GPs in his surgery in Chiswick High Road in London, used a simple intercom system to call patients in to see him. He would read down his long list of patients, find the next one, press the buzzer and call out the name.

On one particular occasion, he noticed the name was rather unusual. Let's say it was Dalziel. A Scottish name and not common at all in the leafy suburbs of West London. After a short pause, the surgery door opened and in came a rather hesitant Mr Dalziel accompanied by his equally uncertain-looking wife.

'Good morning, Mr Dalziel,' began my dad in the usual way. 'How can I help you today?'

'I've a lump in my groin, doctor,' he said matter-of-factly. 'And it's getting more painful as it gets bigger.'

'Let's take a look,' suggested my dad, and asked Mr Dalziel to drop his trousers and pants as he stood in front of him.

'Give a cough. Fine. And another. Fine. Good. You can get dressed.'

The examination was over, the diagnosis obvious.

'Well, you've got an inguinal hernia, Mr Dalziel. Nothing serious, but you'll need to have it operated on and I will send off a referral letter to the Charing Cross Hospital today. An appointment should be sent to you in the next few days.'

'Thanks, doctor, thanks very much,' said the patient, who swiftly turned on his heels and left the room. Rather bizarrely, thought my dad, his wife remained rooted to the spot.

'Did you want to see me as well, Mrs Dalziel?' he added gently.

'Yes please, doctor.'

'Is it about your husband?'

Pause.

'Erm, that wasn't my husband.'

Dad's turn to pause.

'Er . . . who was it then?' he asked tentatively.

'I've no idea,' she said, to Dad's horror. 'I've never seen him before in my life.'

It turned out that, by sheer coincidence, two people with the same unusual surname and who were totally unrelated had booked in to the same surgery session one after the other. Hearing the name 'Dalziel' on the intercom, they had both risen from their chairs and entered the room simultaneously. Neither had uttered a word to the other on the way in and neither said anything to the other in the consulting room either.

Mr Dalziel was obviously quite prepared to drop his kecks in full view of a woman he didn't know from Eve and Mrs Dalziel was apparently quite happy to witness it. Quite what was going through their minds was anybody's guess. Perhaps *he* thought she was a receptionist or practice nurse, despite the fact that she wasn't wearing a uniform. Perhaps *she* thought that examinations of that kind were still sometimes performed in an army-style line-up and, just like mixed-sex wards in NHS hospitals, it was something you had to endure.

In those days the doctor's word was gospel. You never thought to question it. I often asked my dad how he had resolved the issue of the Dalziels. Over boozy Sunday lunches when we enjoyed the fantastic food my mum had prepared, I implored him to tell me what had happened next. But I never found out because whenever I asked, he just fell about in a fit of hysterical laughter.

The thing is, this kind of professional faux pas would never occur these days. Doctors no longer command the same respect from their patients or from members of the public. They used to be seen as pillars of society that people would look up to, admire and revere. These days they are just another state-controlled operative you have to get past in order to obtain your prescription or referral to the specialist.

Not everyone feels like that, however. You still get the occasional old boy who you know has gone to enormous trouble to put on his best Sunday suit and tie to come and see you, and the little old lady who has prepared tea and ginger cake especially to coincide with the house call she has requested. I suppose it is partly a generational thing. But my dad's fantastic story from his days in general practice illustrates the changing fortunes of the medical profession just perfectly.

I often think about my dad, his fascination with medicine and his dedication to his patients. My dad was totally committed to his work as a family doctor and in the early days of his career was often on call around the clock for seven days a week. He was incredibly popular with his patients, who would frequently stop him in Chiswick High Street to chat, and he regularly brought home bottles of whisky or wine that had been presented to him, especially around Christmas time. In those days, a GP's salary was comparatively meagre, so any little gifts like that were always welcome. Once, a patient of his who would now be called a refuse collector, but would then have been a dustman, called in to thank him for the care he'd received over the years, and left a £10 note on his desk as a Christmas bonus. Having a council dustman tip the doctor was both ironic and touching at the same time.

Living in Chiswick (an up-and-coming part of London in the sixties and seventies), Dad had a few celebrity patients on his list, including at one time the quiz show host Eamonn Andrews and one of his comedy heroes, Tommy Cooper, who lived just around the corner in Barrowgate Road. I remember the late Eamonn Andrews ringing up on our home phone one Sunday morning, and since my dad was downstairs in the garage doing his regular keep-fit routine of 5,000 skips without stopping I answered the phone myself.

'Hello?'

'Is your father there? This is Eamonn Andrews speaking.'

'Don't be so silly,' I said and put the phone down. I was only seven after all.

Tommy Cooper was already a legend at that time, and a bit of a local hero. According to Dad, he used to spend quite a lot of time with his thespian friends up at the local pub in Chiswick High Road, where a fair amount of alcohol would be consumed. Also, rightly or wrongly, Tommy had a reputation for being less than generous with his money.

When it was his turn to buy the next round, he would be nowhere in sight. The story goes that on one rare occasion when he *did* buy the drinks, he gave the barman a £10 note and then argued over the change. He swore he'd handed over a £20 note, not a tenner. The barman swore he had received only a £10 note and he even went back to the till to check. Tommy Cooper apparently would not accept this and a heated disagreement continued for about ten minutes. Eventually, with neither side prepared to back down, Tommy took a deep breath, cleared his throat in his unique and characteristic style and uttered the immortal words, 'Look. It isn't the principle . . . it's the money.'

Dad loved sharing his stories about general practice with me and I am sure it had a contributory effect in my choosing medicine as a career. That, and Barbara Windsor in a tight-fitting nurse's uniform, fishnet stockings and stilettos. I admired Dad's diagnostic acumen and commonsense approach to medical problems and I still sometimes find myself in a clinical situation and wondering what he would do in the same circumstances.

One day, for example, I was carrying out a screening medical on a forty-six-year-old man whose father had died at the age of fifty-four from prostate cancer. This was one of the reasons why he'd arranged to have a thorough check-up. I explained that while testicular cancer was predominantly a disease of younger men aged between eighteen and thirty-five, prostate cancer was mainly a disease of older men, with symptoms usually beginning after the age of fifty. I pointed out that one in three men over this age develop symptoms of prostate enlargement, but in nine out of ten cases the cause was benign rather than malignant. The symptoms, I explained, were the same. A weaker stream of urine, hesitancy before the flow starts, a bit of dribbling at the end. Maybe getting up at night more than twice to empty the bladder and a feeling straight afterwards that you haven't completely emptied it. I also pointed out to my patient that a family history of prostate cancer did make screening more important, as there could be a genetic predisposition. I explained that we screen in three ways for prostate cancer: we ask about symptoms, we measure a protein in the blood called prostate-specific antigen, and we do a digital rectal examination using a gloved finger to feel the prostate gland, which is situated at the base of the bladder on the front wall of the back passage. I gave him the consent form that we require patients to sign prior to this test and explained the procedure. I saw the look of hesitation in his eyes, the look that men who have never had a digital rectal examination almost always give.

It's a strange thing. In America, where men are much more health-conscious, if the doctor fails to carry out a rectal examination the patient is likely to sue for negligence. In the UK, if the doctor carries out a rectal examination the patient is more likely to sue for GBH, especially if he hasn't been forewarned. In my medical training it had always been pointed out that the rectal examination was a vital part of any abdominal examination and if it were overlooked the doctor could easily miss an acute appendix tucked behind the caecum, the first part of the large intestine, or a colo-rectal cancer or prostatic malignancy. If you don't put a finger in it, my consultant had said, you put your foot in it. It's a lesson all medical students would do well to remember. My dad would certainly have remembered it and that was why his diagnostic skills were so solid and reliable.

Anyway, one week later the patient who had been so reluctant to have his digital rectal examination (DRE) performed the previous week telephoned me to say how delighted he was to hear that his results were all entirely normal. 'Very reassuring,' he said, and added that a straw poll of his more macho colleagues had come up with a variety of amusing and interesting reactions to the dreaded 'DRE'.

'Do tell,' I said, as if I hadn't heard most of them a hundred times before. What is it that makes blokes such wusses when it comes to a simple medical examination of their bits below the waist? How on earth do they think women feel, whose regular smear tests and other gynaecological procedures are ten times more invasive and intimate than anything a man ever has to endure?

'Well, they came up with a list of everything that male patients having colonoscopies are reputed to have said to their examining physician at the time of the test . . . You know, while the endoscope tube is actually inside the colon and the doctor is looking through it.'

'We call it riding the silver rocket.'

'Ha! Yeah. Something like that. I guess it's because as patients on the receiving end it feels less embarrassing if we attempt to keep up a conversation rather than just lying there and thinking of England. Anyway, number one on the list was "Are we nearly there yet? Are we nearly there yet?" You can understand that one. You can feel the doctor prodding and pushing this bloody metal cylinder up your arse and this strange sensation of fullness and dull aching comes welling up through your innards. You just want it to stop. Number two on the list was "You know, in Arkansas we're now legally married." Next was "Find Amelia Earhart yet?" closely followed by "Any sign of the trapped miners, chief?" ' This was getting better. A couple of these I hadn't heard before. 'Hey, now I know how a muppet feels' made me laugh and so did 'Can you hear me *now*?' The last, 'Hey, doc, let me know if you find my dignity,' was pretty apt.

'Very good,' I finally said. 'Isn't it incredible how blokes find their bowels an endless source of mirth and merriment. The time you really need to worry,' I added, 'is when you're lying on your side curled into a ball with the doctor's finger up your bottom and then he starts nibbling your ear . . .'

'Christ,' said my patient. 'Does that ever happen?'

'Not in my surgery,' I said. 'Nor ever will. Tell you what, though, since you've been so thoroughly grown-up about all this, I promise to write a doctor's note for your wife.'

'For my wife? What will that say?'

'It'll simply say that I carried out a thorough examination of your colon and that despite what she might think, your head is not in fact a long way up there.' This time it was his turn to laugh and once again I thanked God for the value of black medical humour.

I couldn't help reflecting on what had happened. It's curious how a quick, straightforward, consensual diagnostic clinical examination of a bodily orifice could fill most men with such horror and embarrassment. But I suppose the nature of a doctor's job and the sheer regularity of the task makes us professionally inured to it. A doctor, after all, is the only person you can meet for the first time ever who can have his finger up your arse within two minutes and isn't doing anything illegal. Who says the medical profession has lost all its authority now?

Dad would probably be pleased to know that, as a doctor, I can still command at least a tiny bit of respect from my patients but he probably would not be all that impressed with what he would regard as my somewhat frivolous activities in the media. One day, as if to make his point for him, I found myself talking on the Lorraine Kelly show about fashion victims. Hardly the type of hard-hitting medical advice calculated to save lives. Gwyneth Paltrow had been snapped in a very tiny skirt wearing a whole range of seven-inch stiletto heels throughout the week and showing off her magnificent legs. My job was solely to point out the medical pitfalls of trotting about in such unsuitable footwear, although I knew that on the face of it my comments were going to sound boringly practical and dull. So I started by saying how truly sexy any man finds this kind of heel. It is, after all, the very stuff of many men's erotic fantasies – including mine. Lorraine just laughed. I highlighted cases where women had literally toppled off their shoes and either badly sprained the lateral ligament of their ankle or broken the bone right across in what orthopaedic surgeons refer to as a Pott's fracture.

A leggy model ambled down some steps and into the studio to demonstrate the hazard. She was also wearing the very tight silver leggings recently sported by Victoria Beckham, a viciously laced-up corset to emphasize her tiny waist, and a huge but very trendy handbag supported on one beautifully tanned shoulder. Every hot-blooded male doctor's nightmare, obviously. Just imagine the crippling back strain on the creator spinae muscles imposed by carrying such an unbalanced load in that bag. Consider for a moment how the increased abdominal pressure exerted by that corset would interfere with digestion, create uncomfortable wind and exacerbate irritable bowel syndrome or painful periods. Focus on the growing number of women inconvenienced by recurrent vaginal thrush and irritation caused by the constrictive and mechanical friction effects of restrictive hosiery. God, it must be hell being a woman sometimes, I thought, and I spent the rest of the day soul-searching in a turmoil of erotic empathy. It was difficult frankly to get the image of those tight leggings and those oh so impractical, slender but beautifully sculpted seven-inch stilettos under those slim, elegant ankles completely out of my mind. But being the consummate professional I am, I managed to stay in some kind of control. Luckily a boring medical conference was next on my agenda and sitting through a few tedious hours of that soon seemed to knock any remaining images of scantily clad supermodels clean out of my head.

Suitably chastened by dull medical academia, I found myself driving back home from the conference while listening to a late-night radio show where the presenter and his guest doctor were taking calls from the public on the subject of how to complain about your doctor. My ears pricked up.

One irate listener called in and started yelling down the phone, 'I want to complain about my doctor. You can't get to see him. When you do see him, your bum is only on the seat for two minutes. He doesn't look up at you while you're explaining what's wrong and before you've finished he's already written the prescription. It's disgusting.'

The presenter then asked the doctor in the studio to comment. 'Well,' came the reply, 'that sounds totally unsatisfactory. I think you should telephone him immediately and tell him you are not happy.'

'I am,' screamed the man. 'You're my bloody doctor!'

I burst out laughing at my medical colleague's predicament but I couldn't help thinking, there but for the grace of God go I. That's right, I told myself, you are only as good as your last performance. Since I was probably going to be asked about a big medical story the next day, I reminded myself not to let my guard down.

In fact, that week it was the sixtieth anniversary of the NHS. All the TV channels including GMTV were covering it and so were the daily papers which had been running articles on and off for the last few months. I was planning to provide one newspaper with a double-page spread featuring an original and family-orientated board game all about the NHS, based on Snakes & Ladders. The idea was that players would compete against each other to obtain their chosen NHS operation in as fast a time as possible. Throw a six, for example, and you jump the waiting list. Land on the postcode lottery square and you advance at everyone else's expense. Use your union's private medical insurance policy and get keyhole surgery on your gall bladder within days.

Designing the game proved harder than I thought. There were far too many snakes and hardly any ladders. Snakes everywhere in fact, not a ladder in sight. In the game I had devised, nobody would get anywhere near a referral letter from their GP, let alone the doors of the operating theatre. Hospital wards closed by a winter vomiting bug: go back two squares. Operation cancelled due to an emergency admission: retreat four squares. Awake during anaesthesia, go directly to Psychiatry. Consultant still on the golf course, miss a turn. Wrong kidney removed, return to Start and collect a litigation card. It was clear this game would be too depressing and scary, so I decided to shelve the idea. Getting an operation performed successfully on the NHS could never be as troublesome as that, surely?

In the media spotlight I often enjoy a little political rant about the disastrous and ill-advised bureaucratic tinkering the government insists on imposing on the NHS, but some of the most interesting broadcasts are the controversial ones. MMR – is it safe? Euthanasia – should it be legalized? That sort of thing. One of the funniest examples was a debate we planned to have about the pros and cons of hormone replacement therapy (HRT). A newly published medical meta-analysis of thousands of women taking HRT over many years concluded that taking it for more than five years could significantly increase the risk of breast cancer and deep vein thrombosis without offering protection against heart disease, which had previously been claimed. This flew in the face of a previous scientific study which basically said that HRT was effective and safe, especially when used in women with no family history of these two conditions. I was going to say that, for women with mild to moderate symptoms, trying natural alternatives to HRT first was a good idea. I intended to add that, for women with severe symptoms whose psychological and physical discomfort was seriously affecting their quality of life, HRT could dramatically improve their well-being, abolish their symptoms and provide the best possible protection against osteoporosis, one of the biggest causes of disability and death in post-menopausal women.

Opposing me in the TV debate on the sofa was Maggie Tuttle, a fierce critic of HRT in any shape or form and who was due to head up a major conference for women who wished to share their unfavourable experiences of these hormones. When I met her in the Green Room I found her pleasant and engaging but odd. There was just something about her. We went on together in the news hour where she soon made her feelings felt. She considered the pharmaceutical industry to be an instrument of the devil and all doctors prescribing their medicines to be hell bent on poisoning their patients for monetary gain. She went on to catalogue a long list of her own symptoms which she claimed had been caused by HRT, including generalized hair loss and mood swings, two of the very symptoms HRT is reputed to significantly improve. Her accusations were flimsy, non-scientific and subjective. So I said so. The discussion finished after a few minutes, and Maggie and I retired to the Green Room to continue our disagreement in private.

There, over a cup of tea, she said something so extraordinary that I knew I could dismiss her arguments totally if only I could get her to repeat it verbatim in the main programme with Fiona Phillips at 8.10. When the time came I deliberately goaded her with some gentle ridicule. 'Maggie believes that all doctors are evil and that the pharmaceutical industry is immoral and should be wiped off the face of the earth. She hasn't a shred of evidence to support her statements and the forthcoming conference and the publicity it generates will unnecessarily worry women enormously.'

I could feel Maggie bristle beside me. 'Fiona,' she said, 'women write letters to me and tell me what has happened to them. I've got women who've grown penises after taking HRT.'

'How many?' I asked. 'Women that is, not penises.' I felt elated. She had actually gone and said it. Fiona and Eamonn Holmes were almost sliding off the sofa as they tried to contain their giggles yet when pressed Maggie could not provide evidence for her accusation, merely saying that we would have to come to the conference to get it. The discussion ended with Maggie incandescent and me with an amused expression on my face. The duty telephone log was later inundated with calls saying that Maggie had done more to jeopardize the anti-HRT cause in three minutes than any number of favourable newspaper reports over the past ten years.

I have to admit I felt a bit smug. Penises indeed. I don't think so. I don't know where Maggie is now but she's probably taking plenty of red clover, soya bean and linseed as a healthy alternative to HRT. I wish her well.

Talking of penises, which Maggie had been, I couldn't help noticing that in the newspapers that day the World Anti-Doping Agency, which regulates the use of drugs for sportspeople, was reported as considering a ban on Viagra as it was now regarded as a performance-enhancing drug. What kind of performance were they referring to? I'd always regarded this little blue pill as capable of improving sexual performance in men suffering from erectile dysfunction but I found it harder (so to speak) to understand how it could possibly assist athletes on the running track. I mean it's not actually diverting blood to the areas you want it to go to, is it?

Already speculation was rife. Given that athletes have a penchant for wearing extremely tight Lycra shorts, officials would be more likely to notice deliberate doping. But wouldn't the physiological effects of Viagra cause a serious handicap in the hurdles? What if they couldn't get their leading leg over? What about embarrassing confusion in the relay when it came to handing over the baton? Not to mention the pole vault. Obviously any unfair advantage would need to be stamped on hard. Stiff penalties were called for.

Jokes about Viagra – or sildenafil, as it is better known to research chemists – are extremely familiar to doctors. The ointment version of it, for example, that you rub on but then find you cannot bend your fingers for the next three days. The lorryload of Viagra carjacked and driven away by robbers – causing police to go out looking for hardened criminals. It is all very predictable and rather puerile, but still somehow quite funny. A little while ago, however, I found myself talking about Viagra in a sensible medical context for a change.

Four little blue tablets of Viagra were being brandished in

front of the TV camera by none other than Lorraine Kelly. Why? Well, that day she and I interviewed Yvonne Finlayson and Mark Rustan together with their eighteen-month-old twins Ava and Lewis. After several failed attempts to conceive using IVF treatments, they finally went to America to try an unlicensed approach using Viagra. It appears that in many cases of unexplained infertility – where tests have failed to show any identifiable abnormality – the underlying problem is that the lining of the womb is too thin. This means that a successfully fertilized egg cannot properly implant itself into the womb lining and start growing, leading to yet another miscarriage or more infertility. Viagra, working as it does to release chemicals that increase blood flow, seems to thicken up the lining of the womb and enable implantation of the embryo. It is taken not as a tablet, in fact, but as a vaginal pessary four times each day for seven days. Then it is washed out of the patient's body prior to the fertilized egg being implanted as it might be harmful to a growing baby. It had certainly seemed to work for Yvonne and she and Mark were delighted to come on the programme and talk about it.

More research will need to be done to assess just how effective Viagra treatment really is for this condition, but logically there is a good scientific reason why it should work and plenty of grounds for optimism. But as the interview finished, where had those four little tablets suddenly disappeared to, I asked myself as the sound technician divested me of my microphone. Typical. Those guys in the props department had already snaffled them. Not for the treatment of infertility either, I thought.

3

Dead Scary

THE PATHOLOGY MUSEUM IN ANY MEDICAL SCHOOL IS A uniquely eerie place. Tucked away in the bowels of the hospital where members of the public never venture, pickled body parts and sections of human organs dissected long ago float about in clear perspex display cases in a turbid sea of formalin. The specimens within, which are of a grey-brown colour and come in a variety of sizes, fill every inch of space in this vast and strangely silent mausoleum of a room. In this library of death lie the selected remains of countless ex-patients of the hospital who once lived happily nearby with their families, worked in local markets and shops and walked the neighbouring streets and parks until a random abnormality or inflammatory process inside them started to manifest itself as a serious symptom and ultimately claimed their life. The study of such forensic material is not called morbid anatomy for nothing.

Yet despite the ghoulish atmosphere in the room and the disturbing nature of the exhibits, it is a fascinating and enlightening place to be. The ghostly content of each

49

perspex box tells a clear and indisputable story. It is a silent witness to the malignant or degenerative process that either acutely or progressively killed the patient from which it came. Beside it is a painstakingly indexed and laminated library card cataloguing the age and occupation of the donor and pointing out the pathological changes visible which resulted from their underlying disease. As a medical student, I had spent hours in the pathology museum of the Royal Free Hospital studying the morphological changes involved in heart disease and cancer. I had learned more there than from any number of tedious medical textbooks and lectures. There, the specimens spoke for themselves. Even today, I still find it interesting to come back and visit the museum occasionally, to pop into the Wellcome Museum on Marylebone High Street and the Black Museum at Scotland Yard where the work of famous murderers is documented, and the London Hospital Museum where the twisted and deformed skeleton of John Merrick, the 'elephant man', stands bent and contorted in a corner.

The purpose of one visit, however, was very different. With me was sixteen-year-old Dan Jones, the eldest son of some very good friends of mine, Debbie and Adrian. They'd mentioned Dan was extremely interested in pursuing a medical career and was just about to decide which 'A' levels to select at school. As he didn't have any personal experience of medicine and doctoring, I had been more than happy to chat to him about it and had innocently offered to show him the museum, which I hoped would foster his interest further and give him a special preview of what his future medical training might involve.

I had obtained permission from the curator of the museum in advance, and Dan and I were now looking intently at a heart in a jar, massively enlarged by the

50

enormous burden placed on the muscular ventricles by acute narrowing of the calcified and diseased heart valves. We were looking directly at the heart of a patient who had died from the long-term effects of rheumatic fever, a disease all but eradicated in developed countries through the use of antibiotics like penicillin. Even after all this time, scrutinizing these exhibits still had a strange effect on me, and I was acutely aware of how Dan, wide-eyed and relatively innocent at the tender age of sixteen, might now be feeling.

'You OK, Dan?' I asked, wary of any emotional reaction on his part. Even the strongest people sometimes keel over at the sight of blood, and I didn't want my eager young charge upset in any way.

'Yes, fine,' he said. 'It's amazing, really interesting.'

The next specimen was a horseshoe kidney, so called because the two kidneys were fused into a single semi-circular one with not just two urinary outlets draining downwards to the bladder but four. I explained to Dan that of all the congenital abnormalities in the human body, among the most common were those affecting the kidneys and bladder. The urological system begins life as a single duct which separates into two to form the kidneys and ureters. But in a surprisingly high proportion of the population this process fails to develop normally. Consequently, there are thousands of people walking around today with just a single functioning kidney who remain blissfully unaware of it, or only find out if they have investigations for some other condition such as a kidney stone or recurrent infections.

'OK so far?' I gently enquired.

'Yeah, brilliant. Incredible.'

We moved on to the neurology section. Here was a brain containing a huge blood clot resulting from a stroke. Here was a spinal cord transected by trauma in a road accident, and a brain tumour expanding across the cranium to compress all normal structures in its path.

'Still feeling all right?' I probed.

'Absolutely! Amazing!' said Dan. I have to say, he looked genuinely transfixed.

In the next area we scrutinized a stomach riddled with cancer and a section of intestine containing a tapeworm measuring an almost unbelievable 18.5 metres in length. And later, in an especially large specimen case, we came upon a pair of lungs sectioned across the sagittal plane so we could see right inside them, where they were almost entirely invaded by the solid, pale, gelatinous features of a typical anaplastic carcinoma. The victim, aged forty-two, had been a particularly heavy smoker, the catalogue card told us, and the tentacles of this most aggressive form of tumour could be seen reaching out inexorably through the pulmonary parenchyma.

'Yuk,' said Dan. 'Is that really what smoking does to you?'

'That, and this,' I replied, pointing to another lung specimen turned completely black by tar contamination from cigarette smoke. The healthy, aerated, pinker specimen in the jar next to it contrasted with it brilliantly.

'This is what a normal lung should look like,' I said to Dan. 'Clean, clear and spongy. You sure you are OK?'

'Fine,' insisted Dan. 'This is great.'

The next twenty minutes flew by. We had our fill of bladder tumours, liver cysts, thyroid nodules and conjoined twins who didn't survive. We looked at enlarged spleens, pancreatic malignancy and fractured skulls. We saw the horrendous and lethal results of infections such as tuberculosis, meningitis and orbital cellulitis, where something as simple as a stye on the eyelid can spread to the soft tissues surrounding the eyeball and penetrate directly backwards to the brain. Glancing at Dan, I could see he was in his element.

'I find this really incredible,' he said.

And that was when we moved on to the toe. In the smallest specimen jar in the entire collection, here was a single human big toe surgically severed at its base by the pathologist's scalpel. But at the tip was a surprisingly well demarcated black melanoma about 2cm in diameter which had, according to the information provided, gone on to spread through the blood and lymphatic channels of the body to cause widespread metastatic malignant melanoma, and eventually kill the victim as a result. As I digested this data, I suddenly became aware of Dan on my right-hand side swaying at forty degrees to the horizontal. Christ, he's fainting, I realized. The tiniest specimen in the museum had caused the biggest upset. I couldn't even grab him before he smashed his nose against the corner of a shelf and collapsed loudly on the floor in a heap. He was out cold and pale as a ghost. Oh my God, I thought. I'm stuck in a deserted museum of morbid pathology, surrounded by freakish tissue samples, with an unconscious youth who is the son of good friends, and he's totally away with the fairies and twitching rather alarmingly. There was no one around to help.

It's at these times that you hope reflexes will quickly kick in, and at that precise moment I was sincerely hoping that all my CPR life-saving skills would come flooding back to me. I elevated his legs on to the back of a chair, loosened his collar and fanned his face with the largest catalogue card I could find. This was designed to raise his blood pressure and encourage a little more blood flow to the brain. I remember being vaguely concerned about how I was going to explain returning Dan to his parents with a gash across his nose and several minutes of unconsciousness he would not be able to account for. After what seemed like an age but was probably just two or three minutes, Dan's lids started to flutter and he slowly opened his eyes. Unfortunately he still looked as pale as a sheet and I realized that any attempt to stand him upright would be disastrous.

'Just stay there for a while,' I said to him as he looked around uncertainly, mystified as to his surroundings. 'You fainted momentarily, and we just need to wait for your blood pressure to come up a bit.'

Later, as we sat in the canteen drinking ice-cold water and with Dan still looking a whiter shade of pale, he was shaking his head in utter disbelief.

'But I felt fine,' he said. 'I was feeling really great. I don't understand.'

'I do. Your conscious mind tells you one thing, but your unconscious mind tells you something different. You weren't even aware that the visual effect of these specimens and the way your imagination deals with them can have a significant impact on involuntary mechanisms in your body such as blood vessel dilatation, blood pressure reduction and slow heartbeat. You had what doctors call a vaso-vagal episode brought on through emotion.'

'I fainted. Cool,' said Dan. 'Amazing. But why did I faint looking at a pathetic little toe?'

'Because it's so obviously human, I think,' I replied. 'We'd been looking at internal specimens which are just amorphous blobs that could have come from anywhere. But looking at this toe, it's like looking at one of your own. You know immediately this belonged to a person. Someone just like you. Someone who got up in the morning, brushed his teeth, had breakfast, told jokes and went off to work. This was once a fully functional toe. From a regular bloke. Just like you, he'd have cut his nails, enjoyed the feeling of warm sand under his feet on the beach and maybe kicked a football now and again. This made it personal. That's the difference.'

'Who would have thought that among all those other gruesome specimens a single big toe would have made me faint?' Dan asked.

'Hey,' I said. 'Don't knock big toes. A big toe killed Bob Marley in 1981 and another one killed Jack Daniel in 1911. Marley died from cancer and Daniel from septicaemia, both starting in their big toes. Not a lot of people know that.'

I wasn't sure if Dan would know who Jack Daniel was, but I was pretty sure I'd be enjoying one of his liquid products very soon. I certainly needed one.

Soon after, we returned to the museum and spent a further ten minutes looking at some of the tamer specimens, but this time I was watching Dan like a hawk. He was fine. We could have gone straight home, of course, but the last thing I wanted was for him to remember the museum as the place that freaked him out and caused him to faint. I didn't really want him to think of me as the guy who had put him off a career in medicine for life. Going back into the museum was very much like falling off your horse or bike and getting straight back into the saddle afterwards, just to prove you could do it. But Dan rose to the challenge fantastically and was generous enough to thank me copiously on the way home for the experience. His pride, if not his nose, remained intact, and two years on, his parents have, I believe, now forgiven me, especially as his chosen career in rock music goes from strength to strength.

If I myself had long ago grown accustomed to the blood and guts aspect of a medical career, I was still only slowly becoming attuned to the media equivalent. My agent had arranged for me to do an interview with a new and unknown presenter on Channel 4 who was apparently rather unconventional. His name was Ali G, and we had been led to believe he represented minority ethnic groups, doing his best to give them more of a voice in mainstream television. How could I refuse? Everyone now knows who Ali G is and he certainly isn't as he was described to us. But at this time his first series hadn't yet been broadcast and he was still building up his list of unsuspecting celebrity victims of whom he intended to make a complete fool. As he progressed, he famously asked Ann Widdecombe if she'd ever been given a 'pearl necklace', a thinly disguised reference to a rather messy sexual practice involving masturbation and a woman's chest. She, in her glorious naivety, had apparently proudly said yes, adding for good measure how much lasting pleasure it had given her. Several well-known Tory MPs with plummy voices had also boasted they'd given them to their wives.

Ali G had done a pretty good job too on the Bishop of Durham by asking him what Jesus was like. As I remember it, the bishop had thought carefully for a while before answering that Jesus was rather God-like. To which Ali G had responded with a puzzled look and a second apparently innocent question: 'But what did God *do*?' The bishop then stated with some degree of pomp and gravitas that God had created the world. To which Ali G after a beat simply replied, 'And what? Since then he's just kinda chilled?'

None of this interview or any of the similar ones lampooning middle-class professionals too polite and liberal to patronize their poor ethnic brothers or curtail this ridiculous line of questioning had yet been shown. That was why I had not had the privilege of seeing any previous recordings, which my agent would normally have requested in advance. Ali G was not yet the sensation he became. And I was none the wiser. A lamb to the slaughter, to say the least. But where was the man of the moment? The film crew had set up their cameras, lights and sound in my lounge and I was wondering when he would make an appearance and introduce himself.

'He's incredibly shy and nervous,' they said. 'He's sitting in the car outside and he'll only come in at the last minute.'

I regret to say I fell for this hook, line and sinker. Ten minutes later this tall, angular man ambled into my home in the most bizarre costume I'd seen for a very long time. He wore a shell suit, yellow swimming-cap-type headgear, wraparound yellow tinted shades and a goatee beard. He spread-eagled himself on my sofa and began.

'Wot is it like bein a docta?' His arms spread wide with the fourth and first finger of each hand extended and the thumb and middle two fingers flexed into his palms. This was serious rapper style and I was quickly trying to work out what this peculiar blend of cultures was all about. The overall look was a kind of ironic gangsta rap effect with a distinct Anglo-Asian or Middle Eastern influence.

'It has its moments. But I think it's great. Rewarding. Interesting.' A pause for a little irony. 'I mean it's really interesting meeting people like you.'

'Respect,' he said, extending his arm with a clenched fist at the end of it. I automatically extended my own fist to meet his.

'Yo.'

'So is it easy for you as a docta to get hold of drugs?'

'Oh yes. Of course. I just go down to the chemist and get as many as I want.'

Pause.

'Could I get to be a docta?'

'In theory, anyone can, but there is quite a lot of studying to do. Six years of it in fact.'

'Even tho I is black?'

'Why not? There are lots of excellent black doctors and there's no reason you could not be one of them.'

Pause.

'An then I could get hold of drugs?'

'Loads of them.'

'Wot do you fink of pineapples?'

My turn to pause.

'Pineapples? They are a refreshing and tangy tropical fruit containing lots of bromelain which is thought to be useful for a healthy digestion. I like them.'

'But wot about the ones you get from da dealers in da nightclubs?'

Now I had no doubt where this was going, and I adjusted accordingly.

'Call me old-fashioned but I've never really tried that kind. I like the ones that come off the tree.'

Ali changed tack.

'Wot is it like doin an internal?'

Oh wow. What a question. At this point I still wasn't 100 per cent sure this guy was taking the mickey, and I didn't want to make some ribald, potentially offensive joke that might blow up in my face when the media got hold of it. He was very, very convincing. That is why his unique brand of humour works so well, and fools so many people. But I didn't want to come over as a stuck-up, humourless, rude, arrogant, racist pig either. So I carried on cautiously.

'It's a necessary part of a full and thorough examination when the medical situation demands it.'

'I is hearin you. I is hearin you. Respect. But wot if it is a woman?'

58

'Especially if it is a woman.'

'But not if it woz my muvver? She is black and twenty-two stone and lives in a little flat in Tower Hamlets. And coz she's fat, like, she stinks.'

'I'm sure your mother is a charming and lovely lady who you love dearly, and if I was her doctor it would be a pleasure and privilege to look after her.'

'Even though she stinks?'

'Even then.'

'Right. I is hearin you. Respect.'

For two hours, Ali G lolled on my sofa looking gormless and hopelessly ill-educated and crass. He played the innocent and embarrassing social misfit brilliantly. It was a superb act, and his questions had been cleverly thought out and planned in advance. He never allowed himself to slip out of character right up until the time he left. I couldn't help wondering how, if this interview was ever going to be aired on national TV, it was going to make me look. And for that matter, what the ever-watchful General Medical Council was going to think of my answers. Yet all the while during this bizarre inquisition, I must have had a permanent little grin on my face suggesting I knew all along it was some kind of set-up. It just didn't seem to be real. Couldn't be. I may not be the most street-wise doctor on the planet, but I'm not all that naive either. My answers were deliberately over the top and I often found myself laughing out loud at both his questions and some of my own answers. Maybe that was why the interview lasted a full two hours. Ali G wasn't getting the responses he wanted. In retrospect I felt I'd taken the right approach, because apart from a clip lasting a few seconds I don't think the interview was ever broadcast. But I cannot help hoping that I'm not speaking too soon. It could be that Ali G is keeping the best until last, and that I'm in for a horrible shock any time now.

I did not have to wait too long for a harrowing experience of an altogether different kind, however, because at 8.15 the next morning I was lying in bed still wondering whether I was going to be put on the spot again when the phone rang. It was my son's wife, Una, and she sounded upset. Tristan, my eldest son, had been admitted to the Royal London Hospital in the early hours of the morning with what was considered to be either a brain haemorrhage or meningitis. Either way, the implications were horrendous. Una is a highly competent young doctor herself and she would not sound emotional unless there was good cause.

Personally I was in bits already, just hearing the news. I promised to get on a train right away and join her at the hospital as soon as I could.

When I got there ninety minutes later, I found the casualty department filled with a madding crowd of people of every nationality speaking different dialects and being helped by a number of translators each describing their client's symptoms. The staff raced around doing the best they could in difficult circumstances. Tristan and Una were in a darkened cubicle with Tristan nursing a terrible headache and hardly able to open his eyes because of photophobia, but at least he was just about able to say hi.

When I spoke quietly to the consultant in charge, she told me she had not conducted an immediate lumbar puncture as she did not believe from her careful examination that Tristan had meningitis, and she had instead ordered an urgent CAT scan to look for any signs of intracranial bleeding. If this came back normal, she said she would perform a lumbar puncture straight away.

I felt really sorry for Tris. He had developed Type 1 diabetes at the age of seven and had just got on with his life since then, despite having to check his blood sugars on a regular basis every day and give himself four daily insulin injections as well. Yet he was a six-foot five-inch rugby-playing star just about to sit his medical finals and extremely popular with everybody who knew him. Like all my other children, I love him to bits and his gentle laid-back manner is destined to stand him in excellent stead for a successful career as a doctor.

But to date, fortune had not always smiled on him. Apart from Una, that is. They made a wonderful couple who were dedicated to their work and each other.

All of a sudden, the consultant appeared and said that the CAT scan was normal and that she was arranging an immediate lumbar puncture. She carried out her work efficiently while chatting away reassuringly to the three of us. I watched as the three specimens of clear cerebro-spinal fluid dripped into three separate pots and were then labelled with red 'urgent' tags to guarantee their emergency transportation to the lab. Protocol dictates that samples from suspected meningitis cases are processed immediately as with this life-threatening condition seconds count. The samples are duly sent via a hospital porter.

Then we waited. And we waited. And we waited. Nearly two hours passed and still no result. I knew from my work as a patron of the Meningitis Research Foundation that should Tristan prove to have meningitis any delay in receiving the appropriate antibiotics could threaten his life, or at least increase the risk of terrible consequences such as deafness, blindness or paralysis.

As I was contemplating all of this, I heard the consultant on the phone, asking how such a delay could have occurred.

'So where do you think the samples have got to?' she was asking. 'That's not good enough. It is unacceptable.'

As she came back to Tristan's bedside, she was clearly upset herself about the disappearance of his CSF samples and apologized. But it wasn't her fault. For once, I thought that speaking to the chief executive of the hospital could make a difference. I am not one who has ever said, 'Don't you know who I am?' but on this occasion, with my son's health at stake, I was quite prepared to let the powers that be know that someone with potential pull in the media was ready to make a big fuss about the inefficiency of their hospital. The deputy chief executive immediately realized the significance of the call. He expressed his heartfelt apologies and promised to look into the matter straight away, saying that it was important that any such problem was immediately brought to his attention so that he could do something about it for everybody else's benefit in the future.

Interestingly, within five minutes Tristan's results came through. All normal. Would those results have come through had I not made that call? Had it been somebody else's son? As it turned out, Tristan had had his first ever severe migraine attack, a condition which can mimic strokes and meningitis and is often confused for them. He made a gradual but steady recovery and was happily discharged within twelve hours. This was obviously an immense relief to all of us and an experience we would not like to repeat.

I subsequently received an email from the deputy chief executive of the hospital explaining in full the various changes in arrangements for the urgent transportation of samples which he hoped would prevent any recurrence of what had happened. In turn, I reassured him that I only wanted to ensure that constructive comments were taken on board and that I had no intention of taking matters further.

I told him that the staff had done a fantastic job in the circumstances and what they needed most of all was appreciation from patients and their relatives, and a little more support from hospital management.

The day ended on a high when the man in the next bed to Tristan was visited by two large policemen. There was only a flimsy curtain separating the two cubicles in the day assessment unit so we were able to hear every word of the conversation.

'We have got some good news and some bad news,' one told him.

He grunted.

'You have been discharged from the hospital,' said the other.

Another grunt.

'What's the bad news?' asked the patient.

'You are under arrest. You assaulted the paramedic who brought you in last night when you were drunk and disorderly.'

At least it made the three of us smile after a horrible day, and it reminded me of another story about meningitis which I could not resist sharing with my two favourite young doctors to cheer them up further.

One afternoon I had driven down to Bournemouth, where I had been invited to cut the ribbon at the official opening ceremony for a brand spanking new residential home for the elderly. I enjoyed a guided tour of the five-star-hotel accommodation. I was shown the state-of-the-art equipment and all the marvellous facilities that would undoubtedly make any paying guests comfortable for as long as they stayed there. The staff were terrific, the catering first class and, to top it all, the weather that day was glorious. I was ushered into a packed lounge and after a short speech by the managing director I said a few words of my own about how impressed I was by the design and luxury of the building, the qualifications and dedication of the staff and the beauty of the surrounding gardens. I told a couple of little anecdotes involving some of my own elderly patients, which seemed to go down well, and then I cut the ribbon as photographers moved in to take snaps for the local newspaper. Then, as everybody started to drift away, I gave a brief interview to a local journalist before heading for the door myself. On the way, a very genteel-looking lady of about ninety with immaculately coiffured hair and wearing an elegant rose-print dress reached out and took my hand.

'I saw you on the television this morning,' she said in a demure little voice while giving me her most winning smile.

'That's nice,' I replied. 'And I hope you'll continue to watch in the future.'

'You were talking about meningitis, weren't you?'

'Yes, that's right. It's something that we all need to be more aware of so that we can spot any signs or symptoms as early as possible.'

Then she stunned me.

'Is it the black people who brought it to Britain?' she asked.

To start with I thought I must have misheard her. But no, that was definitely what she had just said. There was a rustle of papers behind me as the journalists prepared to scribble down my reply, hoping, no doubt, for some politically in-correct complicit response. The photographer boldly pushed forward, knocking two nurses out of his way. This could be tricky. Bigotry and racism of any kind always appals me but it somehow seems worse when spilling from the foul mouth of some white supremacist lager lout or thug. It was not something you expected to hear from a diminutive and frail elderly lady whose demeanour otherwise smacked of gentility, warmth and compassion. In her case the question was presumably born out of ignorance, the result of ingrained misconceptions developed in an era when immigrants were widely regarded with mistrust and suspicion. But this was one of the first times I had ever heard anybody attribute specific *diseases* to them. Maybe I wasn't all that surprised, but I was slightly taken aback and suddenly very conscious of how my response would be reported.

'W. . .e. . .l. . .l,' I said, thinking fast. I could not agree with her suggestion, but neither did I have the heart or the ruthlessness to chastise her purely for asking what she erroneously and innocently thought was a reasonable question. It did not seem likely that I would be able to dis-abuse her of her very long held beliefs after so many years.

'It's a complex issue, meningitis,' I cautiously began. 'It's caused by a number of different micro-organisms, both viruses and bacteria, which can be passed on to anybody, by anybody, affecting children and adults alike, independent of race, status, creed or religion. It is a universal illness which everyone needs to remain aware of and take steps to protect themselves against.'

The eavesdropping journalist looked disappointed. No scandal or scoop. The elderly lady smiled at me benignly. The photographer was replacing his lens cap. As I looked up, I saw the managing director cock his head in the direction of the exit, a wry smile on his face. It was time to go. And not a moment too soon.

4

House Calls

WHY CAN I NO LONGER REFER A PATIENT I HAVE SEEN, investigated and diagnosed to the hospital consultant specialist I know will be best for that patient? For years, that was what I did as a GP and the practice worked extremely well. If I spoke to that specialist and said it was urgent, he trusted me and would fit that patient on to the end of his list the same day. Alternatively, he might see them on the ward as soon as they could get there. The consultant knew I would not waste his time and the patient's duodenal ulcer or dissecting aneurysm (a diseased major artery which balloons outwards and can rupture at any time) would not have burst open before they could be seen. But today, none of that is possible. All doctors are micromanaged by bureaucracy and now I can only refer a patient to a general hospital department where administrators will allocate that patient to one or other specialist. It doesn't matter how long that might take. Nor does it matter whether that specialist and that patient are likely to get on personally. Nor that the GP and specialist have a good mutual understanding and rapport.

Apparently that is the way it has to be these days. Us doctors have no choice. Computer says no. Shame.

House calls by doctors are managed differently as well these days. General practitioners voted to give up their traditional round-the-clock responsibility for their own patients a few years ago, and the duties were shared out between groups of largely anonymous jobbing physicians teamed up in 'co-operatives'. This led to doctors you had never heard of, never met before, who did not know you or your medical history, coming to visit you on your sickbed or seeing you in some allocated medical centre and sometimes covering a catchment area of 200 square miles in order to make this happen. It was far from satisfactory. But now GPs have had a change of heart. Many now want to take back that responsibility for twenty-four-hour cover and provide proper emergency care for their own patients. Quite right. They should never have given it up in the first place.

When family doctors signed a new contract with the government in 2003 and opted to work from nine to five, it was always going to be a disaster and I said so publicly at the time. The government had no idea how much valuable work GPs carried out in the evenings, nights and weekends, and no practical substitute service was properly piloted or put in place. So almost overnight, sick or dying patients could not get access to a doctor quickly, A&E hospital departments were swamped with people with trivial ear-aches or sore throats, ambulance crews were treated as a glorified taxi service and doctors suddenly found that the most interesting and rewarding part of their job had been cynically surrendered just for an easier life.

It happened for two main reasons. The government had totally underestimated the value of GPs' out-of-hours service and agreed to reduce the doctors' pay by a mere £6,000 per annum. GPs could not believe their luck. They were being told that for the first time since the NHS was set up in 1948, they could clock off in the evening, give up all weekend cover, and after tax be only about £3,600 worse off. All those nights getting out of bed to see people with heart attacks, asthma and seizures were going to be a thing of the past. All those weekends visiting up to twenty patients a day with fevers, belly ache and blood clots – no longer. All that time on the road, finished. All that responsibility and hassle, gone. And all for a few quid. GPs thought they had died and gone to heaven. Especially since a new remuneration scheme for work that they were already doing promised to more than make up for the financial shortfall. It meant doctors could spend more time with their families and less time on the exhausting conveyor belt of seeing one patient after another every ten minutes. Doctors would have been mad not to sign that contract. So they almost bit the government's hand off when it was drawn up and presented to them on a plate.

But now, five years on, GPs are having second thoughts. It has taken five years of patients dying because doctors do not get to them early enough. It's taken five years for doctors to see that nine-to-five medicine is really pretty dull, and that the information gained from seeing a sick person in their own home, in their own environment and with their family around them can be more significant and helpful than any number of visits they might make to the doctor's surgery.

Unfortunately, doctors will not resume doing house calls for the money for which they gave them up. But some of the extra money they were paid to offer 'enhanced services' during the normal working day and which they were already providing and should have always provided *could* be used for the purpose instead. Even then, I'm afraid it will never happen. It is not cost-effective to employ highly qualified doctors to sit in heavy traffic and waste up to one hour visiting a single patient living in some lonely rural location. He or she could be seeing ten patients in the surgery instead. It is not reasonable to ask GPs to make house calls alone at night in some dingy sink estate where gangs would gladly beat them senseless for the syringes, needles and morphine they carry in their medical bags. The old-fashioned house call from the doctor you knew and trusted and who had probably brought you into this world, cut your umbilical cord and helped you later on with your teenage angst, and who knows you through and through and has memorized your medical history, is familiar with your allergic reactions and greatest fears is dead. And so too is general practice as we used to know and love it.

Looking back, I learned a huge amount from the thousands of house calls I must have made over the years. Many people simply wouldn't believe the squalor and misery that some folk are forced to, or sometimes choose to, live in. Many would not comprehend the contrasting wealth and lifestyle of families living just a few miles apart. The challenges presented to a GP acting alone, tired, vulnerable and often in situations of danger were immense, but often very rewarding and satisfying.

In the course of my various house calls, I have probably been amazed, frustrated, angry, shocked and amused in equal measure. It is always good to recall the home visits where I know I made a real difference. The patient with severe asthma whose breathlessness eased dramatically after a slow intravenous infusion of aminophylline. The guy in agony from a heart attack made pain-free and calm with diamorphine. But it still irritates the hell out of me when I remember those house calls in the middle of the night that turned out to be a complete waste of time.

Invariably, no matter what I privately thought of the person who had requested the house call, or the occasionally pathetic or inappropriate reason for doing so, I always tried my best to be polite and professional. Even when I had to get out of my bed for the fourth time on the same night, only to find that the idiot with 'severe abdominal pain' merely had wind. I would calmly reassure him before driving home in a rage. On dozens of similar occasions I have felt equally annoyed, just biting my lip and holding my tongue until I drove home cursing and swearing in frustration and anger, knowing that I wouldn't get back to sleep before the next morning's surgery. There was, however, one exception which broke my habit of always being polite on house calls, and helped me move on in terms of medical maturity. At 1.20am Mr Mathews (not his real name) phoned the surgery's emergency number and was put through to me, the doctor on duty, as I slept at home.

'I want yer to come out,' he started. No introduction, no explanation, no please or thank you. Just 'I want yer to come out.'

'What's the problem?' I replied. There was always a chance that you could deal with a simple problem over the phone. Good telephone advice can reassure the patient and often establish that there is no real reason for a house call.

'It's me son. E's got a terrible eadache. I want yer to come out.'

'How long has he had it?'

'Bout an hour so I want yer to come out.'

'Is he being sick?'

'Nah.'

'Has he got any visual problems?'

'Nah.'

'Does he say he's got any neck stiffness?'

'Nah, nuffin like that. But I want yer to come out.'

'How old is your son?'

A pause.

'How old are yer, son?' Pause. 'Nine'een. I want yer to come out.'

'Have you given him anything for this headache?'

'Like wot?'

'Like paracetamol, Nurofen or aspirin.'

'Nah, didn't fink of it.'

'Has he ever had a similar headache before?'

'Nah.'

'I'd like you to give him two paracetamol now, which might well do the trick, Mr Mathews (not his real name), and then call me again in an hour if it's no better.'

'Aint yer comin out ven?'

'No, not just yet. But I will if he's no better in an hour.'

I put the phone down and closed my eyes. But sleep would not come. It would be just my luck if this lad had had a subarachnoid haemorrhage from a spontaneously ruptured cranial artery. It happens. Not often, but it happens. It would be ironic if one of the rudest, least intelligent and most uncommunicative people I had ever spoken to on the phone had put me off going out on a legitimate and perfectly reasonable house call. I worried. I fretted. I tossed and turned. Until forty minutes later when the phone rang.

'I want yer to come out.'

'No better?'

'Nah.'

I drove to the address he gave me, looking out carefully for the white pillowcase I'd asked him to drape over his fence so I could quickly find the house in the dark in the notoriously badly numbered and dimly lit street. Unfortunately it had already been stolen by the time I got there. I finally arrived at the house and was ushered in to join the chaotic melee of family members, all aimlessly milling around the ground floor of the place, looking gormless. Eight of them were sat in the sitting room where Dave, the nineteen-year-old son, was sprawled out on the sofa with his feet up, watching telly. He did not look particularly ill, but there was no way I was going to take a medical history and examine him in front of all these people. I loudly ordered all of them apart from the dad out of the room. I was going to rule out a haemorrhage or any other serious problem which he or his dad would undoubtedly sue me or beat me up for if I didn't spot it. I was going to have to be very thorough. I decided I'd do this by the book and leave nothing to chance.

'Whereabouts does your head hurt, Dave?' I ventured.

'In the front, ere.'

'Is it constant or throbbing?'

'Dunno.'

'What does it feel like then?'

'Dunno.'

'When did it start?'

'When I came back from the pub.'

Pause.

'Sorry?'

'When I came back from the pub.'

'About what time was that?'

'Bout one.'

'One? And, er, how much had you had to drink?'

'Dunno. Bout twelve pints, somefink like that. No more van usual.'

'Usual?'

'Yeah, but I don't usually get no eadache or nuffin. That's why me dad called yer.'

I proceeded to examine Dave from head to toe. I knew exactly why he had a headache and knew this whole farce was a complete waste of time, but I still did it anyway. Normal pulse. Normal blood pressure. Pupils equal and reacting to light and accommodation. Normal fundus. No sign of raised intracranial pressure.

Cranial nerves intact. All reflexes normal. No neck stiffness. No sub-arachnoid haemorrhage. No stroke. No brain tumour. No nuffink. I solemnly asked his dad to call everyone in the house back into the room. Fourteen people duly filed back in, still looking gormless. I was simmering with frustration, but I was going to enjoy this moment.

'Dave,' I said, 'has been out to the pub tonight and sunk twelve pints of beer. That is a gallon and a half of ale. A bucketload. He's therefore a tad dehydrated and he's got a wee headache as a result.'

I looked around the room for dramatic effect. Sixteen faces stared blankly back as if to say, 'And?'

'At nineteen, *I* used to go to the pub and get bladdered, and I probably drank twelve pints of beer on a couple of occasions as well. I almost certainly suffered for it shortly afterwards like Dave is suffering tonight. But I *never ever* considered calling the bloody doctor out in the middle of the night when I'd got a headache as a result of it, because I would have felt too bloody stupid and too bloody ashamed.'

Fifteen faces blinked at me. Dave didn't because he was already asleep and snoring by now.

'And if *you* or any member of your family ever bother me or my partners in this ridiculous way again, at this ridiculous time of night, for such a ridiculous reason, you can all go and find yourselves a different practice to register with. If anyone will take you on.'

Silence. I closed my medical bag, stood up, strode out of the room and slammed the door behind me without saying another word. As I drove slowly home, I had a broad smile on my face, was laughing out loud and feeling absolutely great. I had been called out on yet another frivolous house call and the whole thing had been an utter waste of time. Only on this occasion I had said so, with complete justification and candour. It felt good to be so honest with patients. I crawled back into bed at 3.45am and slept like a baby.

Whenever I go to my local DIY superstore, I have to drive past a house I once visited as a GP to attend to an elderly gentleman with an acute exacerbation of his chronic bronchitis. It always makes me smile. I had walked up the garden path with my doctor's Gladstone bag in my hand and gently patted the patient's friendly dog as he came to greet me from his sleeping position on the front lawn. The key was already in the front door – no doubt left there by a thoughtful son or daughter – and I let myself in with the dog following faithfully behind me. Calling out the patient's name and announcing my arrival, I heard his greeting from the front room and went inside to find him lying on the sofa. As the dog took up a comfortable position behind me on the sheepskin rug by the fireplace, I chatted to the man about his symptoms and carefully listened to his chest with my stethoscope. The wheezes and rumbles I heard left me in no doubt whatsoever that he had a chest infection and I duly scribbled out a prescription for a broad spectrum antibiotic to which I first made sure he would not be allergic. His son, he assured me, would have it dispensed by the chemist when he called in at lunchtime to see him. Closing my bag and getting up to leave, I could not help noticing that the poor man's dog had deposited a huge pile of poop right in the middle of the otherwise pristine sheepskin rug.

'Oh,' I said with a nervous laugh, 'do you think your son will be able to deal with what your dog has done as well?'

'I'm sure he will, doctor. Except that isn't my dog.'

Pause. 'What?'

'I thought it was your dog. When he followed you in I thought he was yours.'

'I thought,' I said, 'as he was stretched out in your front garden and padded into the house behind me, that he was yours.'

The dog in question would have happily followed me out of the house again, leaving his calling card by the hearth, except that I had at least moved the rug into the utility room for the son's attention later. I still smile whenever I pass that house. It reminds me of the good old days of general practice.

Consultations in the surgery were less impersonal a few years ago as well. You could often have a little bit of light-hearted banter with your patients which would put them at their ease and encourage them to open up a fraction more.

Recently, for example, I popped in to see Aden Curran in the medical assessment unit at the North Hampshire Hospital, where he was recovering from a nasty bout of pneumonia and septicaemia. Aden was one of the first patients I ever saw at Church Grange Surgery where I was a full-time principal in general practice in 1982, and he was one of those patients it was a pleasure to see because he always came in with a saucy joke or two. On the very first occasion I met him, he had all the classic signs of a slipped disc in his back, and sciatic pain radiating down the back of his leg into his foot. He was moving awkwardly and was obviously very uncomfortable. As a self-employed master carpenter, he needed to make a quick recovery and return to work as soon as possible. I gave him all the usual advice together with a prescription for some muscle relaxants and painkillers. As he opened the door to leave, I finally said, 'And remember, don't lift anything heavy.'

'In that case, doctor, how am I going to have a pee?' he replied.

Once I found seventy-six-year-old Mabel Clark sitting in front of me. With one hand she was clutching her walking stick and with the other she was rubbing her swollen, stiff and painful knee. I liked Mabel. Like so many of my other elderly patients, she never complained. She just stoically endured the minor discomfort of her advancing years, and came in with a bright smile on her face, an endlessly cheerful disposition and interesting little anecdotes from her past which unfailingly intrigued and amused me. A quick examination of the joint contour, the range of movement and the slight bony deformity revealed beyond much doubt that she had moderately severe osteoarthritis. The creaking sensation I felt as the kneecap slid erratically over the front of the femur confirmed it.

'I suppose you're going to tell me it's old age,' she said resignedly, aware that this wear-and-tear type of arthritis was the inevitable result of a life of hard, physical work.

'No, far from it,' I replied as tactfully as I could. 'This is merely an early manifestation of diminishing youth.'

At this, a wide, flirtatious grin spread across Mabel's heavily lined face. 'Thank you, doctor. I rather like the way you put that. In much the same way that I like to say that I'm not a spinster. Merely an unclaimed treasure.'

What a great line, I thought, after Mabel had shuffled off down the corridor studying her prescription and leaning heavily on her stick. And why am I always so inspired and delighted when elderly people like her remain so full of life, humour and vitality? It is such a contrast to the endless stream of bored, taciturn, monosyllabic and uncommunicative teenagers who amble into my surgery with hardly an interesting story between them. Certainly not a glint in the eye like Mabel's or even a hint of a smile. But just listen to me. I sound like a grumpy old man. Maybe I'm experiencing a bit of diminishing youth myself.

I never stopped learning new tricks while carrying out consultations. You could read as many erudite medical textbooks as you liked but the unexpected was never very far around the corner and would forever jump up and bite you. Today, most of the people who come to see me in my medical screening clinic for a full physical overhaul are either paid for by their companies or they are part of a population known as the 'worried well' who are happy to pay a considerable sum of money for a service regrettably unavailable on the NHS. So it was unusual that sixty-five-year-old Gracie Irvine had booked to come and see me of her own accord and at her own expense. She had a number of minor concerns which she felt she had been unable to resolve at her own GP's surgery, and the one thing I could provide was a lot more time. We went through the usual questionnaire to begin with, which included any current symptoms from which she was suffering, her previous medical history, any allergies that she might have and whether she was taking any medication. Her answers were clear and concise and it was soon apparent that she had led an exemplary life, always eating a healthy diet, taking plenty of regular exercise and eschewing medication and drugs in any shape or form.

'Have you ever smoked?' I asked.

'Certainly not.'

'And how many units of alcohol do you enjoy on average every week?'

'None at all. I have been a lifelong teetotaller.'

'Any medications of any kind?'

'Likely in my opinion to do more harm than good.'

And so it went on. I conducted the physical examination and between us the nurse and I carried out the usual investigations including blood tests, chest X-ray, ECG, audiogram and eyesight assessment. At the end of the consultation we shook hands and I promised to send the report to her in a few days. One week later my PA at the health screening clinic telephoned to say that Gracie was not very happy with me. Could I give her a call? I duly complied.

'Mrs Irvine?' I said. 'Dr Jones. You asked me to call.'

'Yes,' she said abruptly. 'Your report says that my blood results show abnormal liver function. You say that this gamma GT enzyme suggests I am drinking too much and I should try to cut down on my alcohol intake.'

'Yes,' I replied.

'But I made it quite clear to you, doctor, I do not drink alcohol. I am a teetotaller. I have seen with my own eyes the effect alcohol can have on people and I made that choice many years ago and have always avoided it. I do not know how you could have made such a mistake.'

I was puzzled. Her biochemical liver function tests certainly suggested an excess alcohol intake, but Gracie was protesting vehemently that she never touched the stuff. Hoping against hope, I tried a last resort.

'Mrs Irvine, you do not smoke and you do not drink?'

'No.'

'Is there anything at all that you take for your health?

Any kind of supplement or tonic, grog or concoction of any kind?'

Pause.

'The only thing I take are my precious Bach flower remedies. And I have always sworn by them. They pick me up when I am feeling down, and relax me when I am feeling anxious. I'm particularly fond of Bach rescue remedy.'

I knew a little bit about Bach flower remedies. I had written a chapter about them in my book *What's the Alternative?*. I knew they were based on extracts of certain flowers thought to have some subtle therapeutic effect when taken very occasionally in moments of crisis.

'How often do you take them?' I tentatively asked.

'On the hour, every hour. Why?'

I gently explained that the plant extracts were dissolved in a base that was 50 per cent brandy.

Locum GP work has proved very interesting too at times. Patients in different areas of the county have different expectations of their treatment, live in different worlds and speak with different accents. They even use different language to describe identical symptoms.

It is fascinating to listen to how people express themselves medically, and their explanations as to the underlying cause of their medical conditions are often bizarre. Also, whenever I talk to patients, I am always intrigued by accents. Colloquial language evolves all the time and placing people's geographical background by their accent has long been a particular hobby of mine. Twelve months ago, nobody was saying, 'Do you know what?' before every sentence. Now, everyone is saying it. 'The elephant in the room' is another fashionable expression, just like 'pushing the envelope', 'let's touch base' and 'getting all my ducks in a row'.

How do these new phrases start? Why are they adopted so readily? How do they spread so quickly? I was thinking about this on the M3 driving to work when I saw a message on an overhead digital display screen saying, 'Don't hog the middle lane'. Hog? Strange word, I thought, for the road safety people to use. Not like 'Stay two chevrons behind the car in front', or 'Slow-moving traffic ahead', or 'Gritting in progress' – all sensible, sound, polite. Instead, 'hog'. Isn't this the language of the frustrated motorist cursing, rudely gesticulating and yelling obscenities at the driver who hasn't bothered to move back into the slow lane when others are approaching faster from behind? A French message board would simply read '*Serrez à droite*' – in other words, stay on the right, in their slow lane. Concise, to the point, no slight or criticism implied. Just perfect traffic safety sense and all-round good advice. So who writes the British messages? And what will they come up with next? 'Weaving across lanes is for retards?' or 'Switch your fog lights off, you moron'? It wouldn't surprise me.

Good communication skills are vital for doctors as well. I became aware of just how important they are from my very early days as a medical student, doing ward rounds with the consultant or professor. They would often stand at the foot of the patient's bed with their medical entourage, talking about that terrified person in the bed as if they did not exist. 'This patient clearly has a mitotic lesion in the pulmonary parenchyma, which has extended to the hilar nodes and beyond. We will ask the surgeons if there is any prospect of a total excision, otherwise we will look into palliative DXT. Good day, Mr Bloggs.'

Then they would stroll over to the next bed and scare the hell out of the next patient as well. I often found myself drifting back to see the Mr Bloggses of this world after the ward round, to check if they wanted to know what on earth it all meant. Invariably they were hungry for information and delighted that someone had taken the trouble to come back and explain.

It was not hard to work out that offering an explanation was a good idea. I just had to see the look of helplessness on their faces as they were talked at by all these people in white coats and put myself in their shoes for a few moments.

As a boy of about thirteen, I can still remember my first school medical. I was a little tubby at that age and very conscious of my wobbly puppy fat and blotchy skin. The doctor was in his late fifties with a gruff, abrupt manner and he communicated his impatience and general bad temper brilliantly.

'Undress and put your things on the chair,' he commanded. But I was paralysed with indecision. Things? What things? Did I need to take everything off, or just my school blazer and shirt? In my shyness, I naturally wanted to leave as much on as possible. Yet I had no way of knowing how thorough this medical would be. I dithered.

'Hurry up, boy,' he said. 'For God's sake, how can I examine you for a hernia with your trousers on?'

What was a hernia? I wondered. But I took everything off anyway.

'Leave your pants on,' he grunted. 'It's not a nudist camp.'

Bastard, I thought. All so unnecessary. Why do the job if you don't like it? I knew even then that it didn't have to be that way and I could immediately imagine what a difference it would make if a doctor was nice to his patient. Ever since I qualified, I have at least always tried to be kind to patients and to treat them exactly as I would like to be treated myself. What is so hard about behaving like someone who actually cares?

Not all doctors have natural empathy or good communication skills. Some have to work really hard at it and many these days benefit from the courses in communication skills that have been incorporated into modern medical training. Accents, of course, although fascinating, and capable of enriching the English language, can interfere with good communication too. It is not politically correct to criticize overseas doctors for having strong accents that patients find difficult to understand and it certainly isn't their fault. But if a little old lady cannot grasp what is being said about her condition and treatment, it does not make for a satisfactory consultation.

I have witnessed an old boy of about ninety struggling to understand what the registrar, who qualified overseas, was saying to him in his strong accent from the Indian sub-continent.

'Could you repeat that?' he asked politely.

Same message.

'I am sorry, I didn't catch that,' he said again.

Same message, but louder.

'I don't understand,' came the third and final response from the bewildered geriatric.

What happened? He was referred for an urgent assessment in the hearing aid clinic on the assumption he was deaf. In fact, his hearing was exceedingly good.

Sometimes it is the patient who cannot be understood by the doctor. The phrases people use to explain things can be amusing, as in 'Tommy's little love tube is sore,' or 'Doctor, I've got sick as hell anaemia.'

At other times they can be misleading, as in 'What's up, doc, I am feeling really queer,' or 'It's a terrible case of the heebie-jeebies.'

A patient's accent can be tricky too, even if it doesn't

82

emanate from overseas. Once, when I was on secondment in my GP training year, I went up to a town called Langholm, near Dumfries in the Scottish Borders. The Scottish accent can be particularly broad up there. After doing our morning surgeries, our small group of doctors divided up the house calls and I was sent to see a lorry driver recovering at home from a stroke he had suffered about one month previously. On arrival, I was greeted by his wife, who ushered me into the bedroom where my patient sat in his tartan pyjamas in his favourite armchair, a local malt whisky by his bedside.

'How are you feeling?' I asked him gently.

'Ah'll be honest, Ah wisnae weel tae be fair. Think Ahm on the men though – see Ah can almost stond now be it Ahm a bit skeewif. Ah say brung on next week – Ah'll be up and about and gieng the wife a seeing tae.'

We chatted as best we could about his slow progress, but it was hard going as the stroke had clearly left him with dysphasia. This means slurred speech, caused by damage to a particular part of the brain. I checked his blood pressure and reflexes and carried out a quick assessment of his nervous system. Then, standing up and addressing the patient and his wife together, I announced that I was delighted to see that any residual weakness in his right arm and leg had gone, and that the only remaining handicap from his stroke was his slurred and almost indecipherable speech.

'What do you mean, doctor?' said the wife. 'There's nothing wrong with his speech, there never was. That's the way he normally speaks.'

Oops! I'd have to learn to distinguish between strong local accents and stroke-induced speech impediments in future. What the experience did highlight, however, was the fundamental value of the doctor's house call as a concept and the contribution of the patient's wife in particular. Since learning that salutary lesson, I have always enjoyed the odd bit of locum work. Odd being the operative word.

Not so long ago in the quiet, well-to-do, staunchly Tory part of the country where I was working as a locum, the practice had a strict policy of no telephone interruptions for the doctor while he was consulting with a patient unless there was a sudden emergency. Very sensible. I had just been looking at Mrs Robertson's ingrowing toenail and her son Joe's ruptured but healing eardrum when the phone rang. 'Damn,' I said to myself, 'an emergency.' I picked up and heard the head receptionist inform me that Brigadier Spalding (let's say) was on the line demanding to speak to a doctor urgently. He sounded important. They put him through. After a short pause, the brigadier started bellowing angrily down the phone at me.

'Jones. I've just been discharged from hospital after having my prostate removed . . .'

'And?'

'Well, my wife Constance says I shouldn't be having a gin and tonic so soon after the operation. But I think I could. I mean, what's the correct medical procedure on this, Jones?'

'If you've just had your prostate out,' I explained with a grin, 'I think you should have at least a couple.' Whereupon I heard the brigadier berating his long-suffering wife in no uncertain terms as he slammed down the phone and nearly ruptured my own eardrum. In this particular neck of the woods, this was what constituted a pressing medical emergency.

Later the same afternoon, a lady came into the surgery for a routine smear test. As it was during the school holidays, she had brought her eight-year-old son with her, and sat him down in a corner of the room with a book. As his mummy climbed up on the couch and got ready, he put his book down and asked what she was doing.

'The doctor is going to give me a check-up,' she said.

'What's that wooden stick for?' he replied, watching every move I made and making me nervous. He was only there at her insistence in the first place.

'It's for testing the cells on my womb inside me to make sure I'm well and healthy.'

'Is it like having sex?'

Pause.

'No, Sam, it's nothing like having sex.'

And thank God for that, I thought. If she'd said yes, it would have meant I had been doing two things terribly badly for the last thirty years.

5

Trauma All Round

IT WAS SUNDAY, 10AM. I WAS LANGUISHING IN BED, ENJOYING a rare lie-in, when the doorbell began ringing insistently. When I answered it bleary-eyed, there stood my friend Bob Chapman with a bright red wad of bandage wrapped tightly round his right fist but still dripping blood on to the doormat.

'Had a bit of an accident,' he said. Apparently he had been investigating a problem with his K'archer pressure jet washer and had taken off the outer casing to have a closer look. Unfortunately, when he tried to pick up the machine it was still going, and he had inadvertently put his hand straight into the rotating fan for the pump and shredded his fingers.

'Wondered if you could put my hand back together without me having to queue for hours in casualty.'

Bob was a very good mate indeed and had done some fantastic building work for us in the past for next to nothing. He'd do anything for me, and although I was a little rusty with my wound stitching, the least I could do was to take a look. We went through to the kitchen and draped

Bob's shaking arm over a thick white beach towel to mop up the blood, but even I wasn't prepared for what I saw next. It was as if he had thrust his hand deep inside a liquidizer and then switched it on. The skin of his fingers hung down in festoons. The bright red flesh and silvery tendons underneath had been laid bare. He could bend his fingers, clench his fist and open it up again, and oppose his thumb to each of his fingertips. So no bones broken, at least, and no severed tendons. But it did not alter the fact that Bob worked with his hands all day. He was a chippie, brickie, plasterer and labourer, and general jack of all trades. He was quite literally Bob the Builder, and Sod's Law being what it is he was also right-handed. I inspected the damage for a while longer as cats meandered around the room and various children came to have a gawp.

'Gross!' they said before ambling off with their breakfast bowls. At least I could see they weren't going to grow up to be fainting types. All in all I did not really feel I could help Bob and I said so. This was a tricky job. Fiddly. It would be hard to sew the various strips of skin together in anything resembling a neat and tidy patchwork. Most importantly, I knew that injuries like this required a specialist surgeon with the patient attending for review on a regular basis afterwards in the local hospital's dedicated hand clinic. There could be permanent nerve damage and future contractures from scarring might make normal hand use impossible. I explained this carefully to Bob.

'Sod it,' said Bob. 'You do it. I'll be there all day if I have to go down to A&E on a Sunday.'

'But I really don't think I'm the best person to do this and there could be problems afterwards. To coin a TV producer's phrase, it could all end up in tears and sick, to be honest.'

'Yeah, well, I don't mind that. If you don't mind doing it, I'd like you to.'

So I slowly but rather reluctantly got to work. It felt a little weird carrying out this painstaking suturing over my own kitchen table. On a smaller scale it was rather reminiscent of the appendectomies and guillotine tonsillectomies GPs used to carry out sixty years ago in the comfort of the patient's own home. Using plenty of local anaesthetic and the finest Prolene sutures I could rustle up from my medical bag, I started at one end of one finger and gradually tried to bring the lacerated skin edges together. The first finger took about thirty minutes, but then I got a little quicker and the whole job took just over two hours. It looked terrible. The kids had come in for lunch by now and thought so too. There were tiny little bits of blue nylon stitches and knots caked in clotted blood everywhere.

By now Bob could barely close his fist or bend his fingers, but I really didn't want him to anyway. The last thing I wanted was the entire line of sutures to unravel and to have his fingers split open like a row of burnt sausages. I couldn't help thinking, what have I done? But we bandaged him up anyway and put his arm in a sling to keep it elevated and prevent further swelling. Bob, being teetotal, turned down a stiff drink, but I had one myself and finished his off too. I pressed suitable painkillers and antibiotics into his good hand and told him to go home, rest, leave the water pressure jet well alone and call me later to let me know how he was getting on.

To this day I still have trouble believing Bob has a perfectly good right hand. There might be a wee lack of sensation in a couple of fingertips, but he's still putting up RSJs single-handed, building perimeter walls out of solid rock and fitting out beautiful kitchens. Come to think of it,

I ought to give him a ring as I've got a long list of odd jobs that I need sorting out right now.

If Bob's experience that weekend was not bad enough, reports came in the following day of a man who had accidentally cut off his arm with a chain saw. John Stirling, a keen gardener, had been lopping a few branches off a tree when he slipped and sliced through his arm below the elbow. Amazingly, he calmly walked over to his neighbour's house and sat down talking until the ambulance crew arrived. When they did, they quickly ascertained where the arm might be found and sent the neighbour to retrieve it and place it in a plastic Tesco shopping bag inside another bag containing frozen Cornish pasties to keep it cold. Fourteen hours of careful reconstructive surgery later, and Mr Stirling's arm was beautifully reattached and showing every sign of heading towards a completely successful recovery.

It was an almost unbelievable story made all the more incredible by the patient's apparent stoicism and courage. As the neighbour said, 'He's a brave man. I couldn't believe he didn't faint.' It reminded me of the climber Aron Ralston, who was mountaineering in Utah's Bluejohn Canyon when an 800lb boulder tumbled down the hill and crushed his hand, pinning him to the canyon wall. After six days he had not been able to free his hand, and was slowly succumbing to hypothermia and dehydration. At this point, he made the difficult decision to amputate his own right hand using a multi-tool.

'I kind of entered a slow state,' he said. 'You are just thinking about what is in front of you each second.'

He described how he became totally engrossed in what he was doing but still had the sense to apply a tourniquet to staunch the bleeding when he cut through the arteries.

'When I amputated, I felt every bit of it. It hurt to

break the bone, and it certainly hurt to cut the nerves. But cutting the muscle was not as bad.'

In fact in many cases of major trauma where amputation of a limb occurs, the remarkable resilience of the victim is the most memorable part.

There was Samson Parker, an American farmer who cut off an arm with a penknife in 2007 when it got stuck in his corn picker and the field he was in caught fire following his attempts to free himself.

In another case a kayaker called David Wilson broke his own leg to save himself from drowning. He'd been shooting the rapids of the Kiewa River in Victoria, S.E. Australia, which was famous for its long and winding waterfalls, steep drops and swirling currents, when a submerged log trapped him underwater and held him there. He said, 'It was soon clear that I was not going to come out, so I pushed my upper body up to get the maximum force of water against it and leverage on my legs, hoping they would break. After a while with a sense of relief one did and allowed me to roll out of the boat. I came to the surface and swam into an eddy and was grateful to be pulled out of the water.'

These high-profile examples of major trauma where the victim seems to be able to carry on almost regardless are, on the face of it, astonishing. But experiences of soldiers hideously wounded on the battlefield tell the same story. Clearly, the human body's remarkable response to such threats to life is a relatively common one. Something must kick in to prevent acute collapse or shock in the aftermath. But what is it exactly, in physiological terms, that can apparently protect us and keep us going?

I remember talking to a bereavement counsellor who had been working with the relatives of people who had died in the notorious Bradford football stadium fire. By chance, I had been watching the live football coverage on TV that afternoon and seen the horror as it unfolded. It was shocking to see supporters escaping the inferno as it engulfed the stadium, their hair on fire and their clothes in flames. They appeared to be ambling along, quite unperturbed and as if in a daze. How was it that they were not screaming in agony? How was it that they were not throwing themselves on the ground in a desperate attempt to put out the flames and ease their suffering? This was also the question the relatives of the victims most wanted to ask. They could come to terms with the loss of their loved one, but what they could not accept was the fact that their son, daughter, husband or wife must have suffered so terribly as they died.

What the survivors of the disaster were able to tell the bereavement counsellors and in turn those who were bereaved was a reassuring and fundamental truth about the nature of terrible injuries and trauma. The survivors stated almost unanimously that at the time their skin was being burned, when their clothes were on fire and acrid smoke was filling their lungs, they had experienced no pain or suffering whatsoever. It was only subsequently, as they lay recovering in a hospital bed and facing the prospect of skin grafts and slow rehabilitation, that the emotional and physical pain started to hit home.

It appears the human body has a primeval protective mechanism capable of blocking out the sensation of pain in moments of crisis. Part of it is the 'fight or flight' response, where noradrenalin and adrenalin create dramatic changes in the body to endow us with enormous strength and power. Another part is the equally spontaneous release of endorphins in the brain. These are potent chemical neurotransmitters similar to morphine and which are capable of creating an anaesthetized euphoria-like state, making us oblivious even to the most acute pain and suffering. The survivors' testimony proved extremely helpful in enabling many bereaved relatives to accept more readily what had happened and move on emotionally. And it also explains how John Stirling, Aron Ralston and others like them who have lost limbs and fingers in industrial accidents can so stoically pick up their bloody amputated limb and carry it to the nearest point of help for surgical reattachment.

However much we may rationalize pain and suffering and try to make sense of it, when we hear news about serious illness in celebrities and people we think we know it still has the power to shock. Few of us could believe it when the news broke about Severiano Ballesteros, the golfing legend who underwent an emergency operation for cerebral oedema forty-eight hours after a brain tumour was removed. The original surgery had caused the brain tissue to swell, and when that happens within the confined space of the skull, increased pressure can lead to loss of consciousness, permanent brain damage and even death unless it is decompressed. That requires a craniotomy, where part of the skull is removed, and medication to minimize further swelling. It was incredible to think that this was happening to the popular fifty-one-year-old Spaniard who had won five majors and eighty-seven titles overall, and captained the side which wrested the Ryder Cup away from the Americans in his home country in 1997.

Brain tumours are in fact more common between the ages of sixty and seventy, but they are frequently seen in younger adults and some occur in children. They can be cancerous or benign, but unlike many tumours in other parts of the body, either can be equally serious depending on its size, location and rate of growth. Such tumours can compress nearby tissue and cause raised intracranial pressure, leading to symptoms such as a headache which is more severe in the morning and worsened by coughing or bending over. There may be blurred vision, nausea and vomiting, unsteadiness, double vision, numbness and weakness of the limbs on one side of the body, and slurred speech. Seizures may occur for the first time, and personality change may occasionally be the first manifestation.

Looking back over the years, I have looked after lots of patients with primary or secondary brain tumours, and none of them was ever easy or straightforward to treat. But I shall always remember one particular case because the circumstances were quite exceptional. It was near the beginning of my medical career when, one weekend at the Royal Free Hospital, while 'on take' for new emergency admissions, I transferred over from the medical post I had occupied for the previous six months to start my new surgical house job. My new post was based on Moore Ward, the oncology ward, where all the thirty or so patients were being treated for cancer of various types and its consequences. Many were very ill or dying, and our role was to make what little life they had left as comfortable as we could. It was a Friday, and wherever possible we would always allow inpatients to go home for the weekend to their families, provided, of course, that they were well enough, tolerating their treatment and not experiencing any nasty side effects. I was doing a final ward round of the day with a very junior nurse and came up to Hamish McDonald's bedside.

Hamish was a huge, stocky, toothless Scotsman who had been transferred over from the surgical unit only two days previously after undergoing a craniotomy for the removal of a frontal lobe brain tumour. The tell-tale surgical scar on his shaven head was still fresh and prominent. I had not yet had time to familiarize myself with his case notes, but he was tolerating his treatment well, and was generally perky and cheerful.

'I don't suppose I can go home for the weekend, doctor?'

'Well, let's see,' I said. 'All your observations are stable, and you're fine with your medication.'

'Are you serious, doc?' He grinned, surprisingly excited by the prospect.

'Where will you stay?' I asked Hamish.

'With . . . with my girlfriend,' he stammered, sitting bolt upright in bed, amazement etched all over his face.

'And you'll be back first thing on Monday morning for your treatment?'

'You can count on it.'

'Then you can go,' I said.

At this, Hamish leaped from his bed, did a little Scottish dance across the floor, grabbed the nurse by the waist and waltzed her round too, then threw on his clothes and dashed from the ward before anyone could say goodbye. Strange, I thought, but gave it no further consideration until Sunday, two days later. As the weekend progressed and our medical team admitted more and more patients from casualty to medical and surgical wards, we carried out an appendectomy here and a laparotomy there, until reaching the point of exhaustion. I can distinctly remember a moment when my registrar and I were doing what we hoped would be a final post-operative ward round just after midnight, when one of the senior nursing sisters came running up to tell us about a patient's significantly raised blood pressure.

'I'm worried about Mr Samuels,' she said. 'His blood pressure keeps going up.'

'So stop taking it,' said my registrar. 'Just stop taking it, then you won't have to worry any more.'

It seems almost negligent now to admit it but we were out on our feet after being on call for thirty-six hours without sleep, and both of us felt some things just had to wait if we were going to function at all. Some time later, after a snatched few hours' kip, I sat in the doctors' room on Moore Ward in the early hours of the morning leafing through some of the patients' notes. Among them were Hamish McDonald's as I felt I really ought to catch up on his medical history.

The notes were about three inches thick, well thumbed and fully documented, but looked no different fundamentally to any of the other patients' records. At the front were his personal details – name, age, address, sex, date of birth. Then there were the medical notes from his original admission onwards, and the surgical notes with details of his operation and treatment. Towards the end, I found the latest annotation describing his current status and neurological findings, and the scribbled note I had added two days previously discharging him from the hospital for the weekend. When I turned over the final few pages, however, I came across a document I had never seen before and hope never to see again. It was very official-looking, headed 'HM Prison, Wormwood Scrubs', and signed at the bottom by the Home Secretary himself. It read: 'Under no circumstances may Hamish McDonald be discharged from hospital without the express permission of the Home Secretary.'

Oh my God, I thought. What have I done?

As I read on, it all became clear. Four months earlier, Hamish McDonald had taken an axe to his landlady's head and killed her. He was a convicted murderer, a dangerous butcher and a homicidal maniac. And I, Dr Hilary Jones, newly qualified junior doctor, had blithely let him out of hospital two days before to go and kill at random throughout London. I froze. I sweated. I shook. What could I do? I didn't know. Should I call my consultant, Dr Boesen, and confess what I'd done? What was the point? What could she do? Should I call the police? Where would they look for him? Was he still protected by medical confidentiality anyway? Was Hamish still a danger to the public, having had his surgery? I wrestled with these questions and was grateful that my general exhaustion at least numbed my anxiety and embarrassment to a significant extent.

But then, look, I reasoned to myself. Could it not be the case that Hamish, of previous sound and unblemished character, had developed a brain tumour in his frontal lobe (as I read he had) which caused his personality to change (which it had done), which drove him to attack his landlady when the balance of his mind was unhinged (this was supposition), and that now he'd been treated he was of no danger to anyone (this was pure hope)? Yes, I decided. I'd sleep on it, and then commit suicide if Hamish didn't return as promised on Monday morning. Suffice to say, I didn't sleep very much that Sunday night, and was mightily relieved when Hamish, with a huge grin on his face, strode up the corridor to greet me at the nurses' station at 8.30 prompt on Monday morning.

'You didn't know, did you, doctor?'

'No.'

'Are you pleased to see me?'

'Delighted. Did you behave yourself, Hamish?'

'You mean did I kill anyone? No. I'll tell you what, now we've established a precedent, if you're free at lunchtime I'll take you over to the Roebuck and buy you a malt whisky.'

I had that whisky with him later, and several others over

the following weeks as he continued his treatment before being escorted back to the Scrubs by two burly uniformed officers. He gave me a huge grin and a wink as he looked over his shoulder when he left. I never heard from him again, but I often wonder what he might now be up to.

6

The Out-takes

WHEN I THINK ABOUT IT, I HAVE ALWAYS PREFERRED LIVE television interviews to anything pre-recorded or endlessly rehearsed. With film on tape there is never the edge you get with live TV and it always takes so much longer to do all the close-ups, cutaways and distant shots that need to be done separately. This is so that the editors can cut up the film later to make it look polished and more detailed. It's all very well making it seem like you've had three different cameras at the location rather than just the one, but it can be frustratingly time-consuming, especially if you are working with a perfectionist producer or cameraman or both. By comparison, what you get with live TV is every little nuance, every pause, every hesitation, every nervous laugh and every darting glance at everyone else on the sofa, as if to say, 'Hey, guys, help me out a bit here will you.'

Live phone-ins are more challenging and fun for exactly the same reason. We were doing one of our routine medical phone-ins on the subject of palpitations one day, and we wanted to cover all the commonest problems people encounter, such as extra heartbeats, missed beats, a racing heart for no apparent reason, and those strange fluttery sensations people get in their chest which make them worry because they think they may be having a heart attack. As is customary for this kind of thing, our producer had already sifted through some of the earlier calls that seemed suitable and lined up a few of them to ring back for me to talk to on air. They'd all been briefed about keeping it short and concise and restricting it to just one specific question. So on this programme at least I had a rough idea of what our callers were going to ask. But you're still never quite sure how they are going to phrase their question, and while they are asking it the camera is centred on me alone. The director, meanwhile, was helpfully exhorting me to look concerned and sincere – as if, unlike an actor simply playing a role, I wouldn't anyway. The first three callers asked why drinking lots of coffee causes palpitations (caffeine is a cardiac stimulant), whether irregular heartbeats signify heart disease (only rarely) and whether it's true that you can stop a heart beating rapidly by pressing hard on your eyeballs with your thumbs (yes). Easy. So far so good. It was all going very nicely.

Unfortunately the fourth call did not go quite to plan. The caller initially asked me about her palpitations and the fact that she only got them when she was anxious or excited. So I reassured her that this was what the stress hormone adrenalin was designed to do and offered the additional titbit of information that palpitations which disappear with physical exercise are almost always benign and harmless. Great. She was happy. Then she hit me with an additional and totally unexpected secondary question about her son.

'While I'm on the phone,' she said, 'I'd like your advice on my eleven-year-old boy who has just been diagnosed with

Spielmeyer-Vogt-type neuronal ceroid lipofuscinosis. Our doctors seem really clueless about it, and don't seem to be able to tell me anything. James is really upset by it and I'm just so grateful you'll be able to fill me in on everything I need to know.'

A great hush descended on the studio at this point as all eyes swivelled towards me, awaiting my brilliant response. Unfortunately, I'd never even heard of lipofuscinosis, let alone Spielmeyer-Vogt syndrome. As it was a term based on the names of the doctors who originally described it, I could hardly even guess at which part of the body it affected. It wasn't perhaps surprising since the condition is as rare as hen's teeth and the average GP would have to be in practice for about 10,000 years before coming across a single case – as I subsequently discovered. But James's mum had 'bigged me up' on live TV and was eagerly anticipating my learned and erudite reply. So were Lorraine Kelly and about two million viewers. On top of that, the director was now also yelling into my earpiece, saying that time was running out and I needed to keep the answer short. Great.

Usually if I'm stuck for a bit of esoteric medical information, I have time to read the books, surf the net or contact a mate who specializes in the subject. It isn't like *Who Wants to Be a Millionaire?* where you can ask the audience. And with anything medical, you certainly can't gamble with a 50:50. But you can phone a friend. Unfortunately, on this particular occasion I couldn't do that either. For a moment time seemed to stand still, then I thought of a way out. I looked directly into the camera lens, using my most concerned and sincere expression. The director would have been proud of me.

'Spielmeyer-Vogt syndrome is a very rare condition indeed,' I said gravely. 'And such a complex and sensitive one that it merits a much more personal and lengthy chat than this short programme today can offer. I'm going to make a promise to you right now because we're running out of time as well: my producer is going to take your telephone number and I'm going to call you back personally after the programme and tell you all you want to know about James's condition.'

In the studio you could hear a pin drop. James's mum was delighted, and Lorraine said what a nice gesture she thought that was. And I'd even managed to sound as if I knew what I was talking about. I was hugely relieved to be off the hook without having made a complete prat of myself.

'I haven't got a clue' isn't, after all, the response you want from a top TV doctor, is it? Ten minutes later, after a fast and furious review of the medical literature on lipo-fuscinosis, I had a long and interesting and, I hope, much more helpful telephone conversation for real with James's mother.

I was highly amused one afternoon to hear about a rival media doctor's disaster on Sky TV. A bit of a newcomer to the scene, he had apparently been asked to come into Sky TV's studios in Isleworth that morning to be interviewed by one of their top news presenters. Arriving a little late as the limo that had been sent to collect him had initially gone to the wrong address, he was quickly greeted before being bustled into the make-up room and then straight into the studio without a further word being said. As he was ushered in, he saw the presenter frantically turning over the pages of her script and looking rather disorganized. She barely glanced up as the floor manager seated him in the chair opposite her. At that moment, the red light on top of camera one came on, and the presenter's posture and facial expression hardened as live transmission began.

101

'How vital,' she began, 'will the role of Hezbollah prove to be in the struggle to find lasting peace in the Middle East?'

The doctor apparently looked terrified and gulped audibly.

'I . . . I don't really know,' he blurted out. 'I'm here to talk about the female condom.'

Just imagine how the presenter must have coped with *that*. The two stories are hardly seamlessly linked, are they? Personally, I am often reminded of the time we were filming a series to teach basic first aid. We wanted to demonstrate what to do if someone had fallen off a ladder and was unconscious on the ground. So at my house we stood a triple-length ladder up against a wall and persuaded my carpenter friend Aden to lie beneath it playing dead. I started my piece to camera. 'If you find a tradesman in this situation . . .' I said, and for some reason then stopped to do a retake. Since we would be doing it all over again, I then added as a joke, 'you can easily hire another one through Yellow Pages.' Unfortunately, it wasn't a pre-record at all and the whole thing had gone out live. I was lucky, though, and we only attracted a couple of complaints from indignant tradesmen's wives. Personally, I'm sure I would have made a lot more cock-ups without the guidance of experienced producers like Michelle Porter. But even Michelle herself has been caught up in TV mayhem before now. She is one of GMTV's best-loved and most experienced producers and has so far always declined the offer of pro-motion to managerial roles, as her greatest interest lies in travelling the world and being involved in the day-to-day making of good telly. It is no coincidence that some of the best and most exciting trips I have ever been on have been set up and organized by Michelle.

Some jobs, by their very nature and sensitivity, require a producer who really knows what they are doing, and the arranged interview between a family caught in the credit crunch and the Prime Minister, Gordon Brown, at 10 Downing Street was one such example. Michelle was ideal for the role. As it happened, her elderly grandmother, Violet Knott, had been admitted to hospital the week before the interview was due to take place. Slightly confused and dis-orientated after a surgical procedure, Violet was delighted when Michelle went to see her and thrilled to hear that she would be visiting 10 Downing Street and producing the Prime Minister, of all people, the following Monday. Who wouldn't be?

Unfortunately, after Michelle had left, Violet made the mistake of telling the nurse.

'She's going to see the Prime Minister on Monday, dear?' said the nurse in the most patronizing tone she could muster. 'Yes, yes, of course she is.'

'At Number 10 Downing Street, no less,' added Violet proudly.

'Where else?'

'Mr Gordon Brown himself, mark you.'

'Well, of course, Violet, I am sure the Prime Minister has nothing better to do with his time than drink tea on a Monday morning with your granddaughter.'

And then, shouting over her shoulder to the nurses' station, she yelled, 'Christine, you had better ask the psycho-geriatricians to visit Violet. She's obviously confused and delusional.'

It was perhaps not surprising that what the elderly lady was saying seemed far-fetched. NHS hospital wards are full of old folk with varying levels of dementia and delusions of grandeur featuring well-known personalities. So it was much to the staff nurse's surprise that on the following Monday morning, when she was making the old lady's bed, up popped the Prime Minister on GMTV with Michelle in the background, just as her patient had predicted.

'That's where my granddaughter is now,' said Violet matter-of-factly. 'Producing the Prime Minister on television.'

But whether the staff nurse had heard her or not was uncertain. She had rushed off to the nurses' station to cancel the psycho-geriatricians' referral.

It often occurs to me when I think about some of the things we do on live TV that we wouldn't be doing them at all unless we were being filmed. Just look at the disastrous stunts they try to get away with in *You've Been Framed*.

Presenters are no different. As long as they know millions of people will be watching, they are quite happy to throw themselves out of planes, bungee-jump over rock-strewn ravines, swim with sharks and eat scorpions-on-a-stick. It always looks good, the action is laid down on DVD for posterity and the TV company pays for the insurance in case anything goes wrong. Everyone thinks you are really brave and the adrenalin rush is incredible, so I can understand how people are sucked in. But it is harder to comprehend why apparently normal volunteers become embroiled in less dramatic and even rather mundane stunts.

Not so long ago there was yet another scare story in the news about the carcinogenic properties of bacon and over-cooked sausages. I drove down to Canning Town to meet our news team in a greasy spoon diner called George's Café in Rathbone Market. TV producers always like to have a bit of visual action going on in the background to illustrate a news story, so Big Dave, as we'll call him, was provided with a full English breakfast, at our expense, and invited to tuck in. As he ate his bacon, sausages, fried bread, beans, tomatoes, eggs, black pudding and potatoes, I talked through the latest research, which suggested a link between the nasty little free radical molecules in cooked fatty meats and cancer. That hit went out at 6.15am. We repeated the hit at 7.10am and again at 7.55am when another story collapsed because of a signal failure on the satellite truck. Each time, Big Dave was provided with a fresh plate of breakfast and each time he devoured it.

It looked really good on TV, the folks back in the studio kept assuring us, so since Big Dave wasn't exactly complaining we carried on. In all, he consumed five breakfasts that morning, all in the name of television, and while it made *me* feel a trifle queasy, I am pleased to report that he has not, to the best of my knowledge, yet contracted cancer or had a heart attack. Maybe that is a news story in itself.

7

Life and Death

FOR MANY, MERCY KILLING IS AN UNTHINKABLE CONCEPT. For some, it represents the bravest, kindest, most loving gesture it is possible to offer someone you care about. For others, it is nothing short of premeditated murder. I can think of no other ethical dilemma in medicine capable of evoking such widely differing and polarized views among the general public.

In October 2008 the issue was once again brought to the public's attention when the mother of a twenty-three-year-old rugby player, Dan James, who killed himself at a suicide clinic in Switzerland, was questioned by detectives investigating his death the previous month. 'WE HAD TO HELP OUR PARALYSED SON DIE' ran one headline, accompanied by pictures of the family taken when Dan was a fit, healthy rugby-playing lad with a bright academic and sporting career mapped out ahead of him. It was extremely difficult to many people to understand how such a young person could possibly have the desire, conviction and courage to take his own life.

Yet personally, when I read the article, my first instinct was to pick up the phone to Dan's parents and tell them how much I supported them in what must have been an incredibly hard decision. How could anybody even begin to imagine the heart-rending anguish that Mark and Julie James must have gone through when their son asked them to help him die. After a rugby accident the previous year had left him paralysed from the chest down, he had no function in his hands, was incontinent, experienced uncontrollable spasms in his legs and upper body and needed twenty-four-hour care. For somebody whose entire life had been centred on physical activity and who had embraced serious dreams of a career as a professional player, it must have felt like a fate worse than death. Who can possibly imagine what discussions must have gone on between them as a family before they came to the conclusion that no medical treatment, no psychological counselling and no amount of round-the-clock care could ever remedy this unacceptably painful and miserable existence? Who, other than loving parents in this tragic situation, could possibly imagine what it must be like to realize that this was the time to grant your son his wish to say goodbye to you for ever? To love somebody that much and to deprive yourself as a parent of their existence in your own life must be the cruellest, harshest, most impossible decision anybody can ever have to make.

In a statement they issued through their solicitor, Julie and Mark said, 'His death was an extremely sad loss for his family, friends and all those that care for him but no doubt a release from the prison he felt his body had become and the day-to-day fear of his living existence. This is the last way that the family wanted Dan's life to end, but he was, as those who knew him are aware, an intelligent, strong-willed and, some say, determined young man. Over the past six months he constantly expressed his wish to die and was determined to achieve this in some way. He was not prepared to live what he felt was a "second class existence".'

To add insult to injury, the Jameses' actions in relation to Dan's decision were criticized by a 'well-meaning' person who alerted the police to Dan's case. Julie James said, 'This person had never met Dan before or after his accident, and obviously gave no consideration for our younger daughters who had seen their big brother suffer so much, and the day before had had to say goodbye to him.'

Julie and Mark took Dan to the Dignitas Clinic in Switzerland, and had to watch while he drank a milky barbiturate cocktail which sedated him, slowed his breathing and finally allowed life to leave his body. This was a decision made by Dan and his parents, and in the circumstances I passionately believe that it was theirs alone to make. What right does any other person have to tell a family like this, tortured by their own grief and suffering, that their loved one should continue to exist in terror, discomfort and indignity?

Once again, the case highlighted the legal and ethical debate over euthanasia in Britain, and Britons who journey abroad to die in countries where it is legal. Under the 1961 Suicide Act, killing oneself is not actually illegal in Britain, but anyone who 'aids, abets, counsels or procures the suicide of another' could face fourteen years in prison. Just a fortnight prior to Dan's story hitting the headlines, multiple sclerosis patient Debbie Purdy, aged forty-five, had gone to the High Court in an effort to persuade the law to make clear the circumstances under which someone could be charged with aiding the death of a terminally ill person. She hoped she would be able to travel abroad to end her own life when her discomfort and pain became unbearable.

With thoughts only of her husband, Omar Puente, in mind, she wanted to ensure he would not be prosecuted if he helped her to travel to a clinic like Dignitas. Predictably, she lost her landmark legal case, with the High Court sympathizing with her but ruling that only Parliament could effectively change the law in this way. To date, more than a hundred people from Britain are thought to have made the journey to the Dignitas headquarters in Zurich, where the slogan is 'Live with Dignity, Die with Dignity'. Switzerland's more liberal laws on assisted suicide mean that prosecution will only occur if people aiding and abetting a suicide are acting out of self-interest. All specialist staff who work at Dignitas are volunteers, which ensures there is no conflict of interest. Yet even there, a national referendum planned for 2010 may very well restrict the practice to the terminally ill rather than people in Dan James's situation, and might prevent non-Swiss nationals from being helped. To date, I am pleased to say, nobody has yet been prosecuted for assisting a death at the Zurich euthanasia clinic.

Yet in Britain the threat in the 1961 Act of up to fourteen years' imprisonment for assisting suicide is ever present. Not just for relatives, but for doctors and nurses also. In all my medical experience, I have found that no two patients are the same, no set of circumstances exactly alike. If I stand by and watch a patient writhe in agony with an incurable and progressive illness, am I a good doctor? If I give pain relief in a form which, as a side effect, will depress breathing to the extent death may arrive a little earlier than nature intended, am I a killer? Is this euthanasia? Is this murder? Let us be clear on what is legal now. There is a very fine line indeed between passively allowing a patient to die and actively bringing about someone's death. Passive euthanasia is legal. Active euthanasia is not. Somewhere in the middle is that vast, uncertain territory that defies definition. It is a kind of ethical no-man's-land.

To what extent do the treatments we use each and every day to control pain, anxiety and suffering hasten the moment of death itself? All doctors have given morphine to terminally ill patients, and morphine always depresses breathing. It is a known, expected and sometimes sought-after side effect. So it could be argued that, to a degree, all doctors perform euthanasia. But isn't the alternative worse? Physicians so remote and callous that fear of legal recrimination overcomes their duty to put the needs and the care of their patients above all else? Increasingly rigid legal guidelines and precise definitions of what doctors can and can't do would put an end to medical discretion. It would be black or it would be white. But there would be no room for manoeuvre.

This is what some people are aiming for, of course. Pro-life campaigners may be incensed by what has happened to Dan James. They may compare his case to that of Matt Hampson, who was also left paralysed from the neck downwards, breathing through a ventilator and relying on a team of carers to bathe, feed and dress him after a similar accident in a rugby scrum which collapsed on top of him. In a national newspaper a few weeks after Dan's case, he wrote an incredibly moving interview about the choice he had made to 'get busy living'. He himself had met Dan, understood his circumstances and declined to comment on whether Dan's decision was right or wrong. Clearly it was right for Dan. As Matt writes about the difficulties in his own current life, he talks positively and optimistically about what he can still do and what he hopes to achieve in the future. He writes a regular column for his local newspaper, coaches youngsters at his previous school, and watches most of the rugby matches at Leicester Tigers.

Some pro-life campaigners and religious groups may feel that there is never a case for mercy killing in any shape or form, and that anybody assisting, aiding or abetting should be prosecuted. They talk about how any medico-legal protocols could be abused, how psychiatrists could treat the depression in patients who are contemplating suicide and how any change in the law would be the slippery slope to mass killing. But there are no doctors running around haphazardly knocking off handicapped babies or confused elderly folk, and there never will be. This would be no charter for people like Dr Harold Shipman, who acted alone and was nothing more than an out-and-out murderer. There is no sinister new medical movement intent on culling the weakest individuals from our society, and callously slaughtering on a whim those born into the world with physical differences. Quite the reverse. I can certainly understand the hurt felt by, for example, cerebral palsy sufferers who angrily say, 'That might have been me they were killing,' but there has never been any suggestion that they might become targets of euthanasia.

Tragically there will always be patients who face a lingering death with protracted periods of relentless and agonizing misery beforehand. How well I remember interviewing beautiful, intelligent and glamorous Annie Lindsell as she was embarking on her own court battle for the right to die with dignity. I had been invited to her home in the suburbs of London to talk about her case, and it proved one of the most moving interviews I have ever been involved in.

Suffering with motor neurone disease, one of the cruellest diseases known to man, all she wanted was permission for her doctor to intervene and administer diamorphine without fear of prosecution. And she wanted this to happen if her condition deteriorated sufficiently to make her suffocate or choke to death when swallowing became impossible, even if it might shorten her life. It is, in fact, a practice that happens day in, day out across the country with the tacit understanding of doctors, patients and their immediate relatives. As I talked to her, Annie was surrounded by those she loved most, was immaculately dressed and made up, was happy and smiling and generally full of life. She even played the piano with her partner as she chatted so courageously about her future. Ultimately, she withdrew the legal case in October 1997 after establishing the principle that doctors could legally administer life-shortening drugs for the relief of mental as well as physical distress. She was assured that her doctor would not allow her to suffer unnecessarily, and a treatment plan was drawn up based on best medical practice.

The Voluntary Euthanasia Society subsequently said that as a result of the ruling, the law had been clarified on passive euthanasia and there had been a step in the right direction for legislation on active euthanasia, where a doctor intervenes to end life when a patient is in a great deal of pain. Motor neurone disease is ruthless. It destroys the nerves that enable people to control their muscles while leaving the senses unaffected. Insidiously, paralysis creeps up the body from below, rendering people immobile and incontinent before affecting their breathing and swallowing. All the while, they know exactly what is happening, and are conscious of the fact that there is no treatment. They can only wait in fear of what approaches.

As it happens, Annie died without recourse to the treatment plan and is now at peace. She was a brave, amazing and beautiful lady and I for one will not only never forget her as a person, but continue supporting her dying wish to win the right for people to die with dignity. Personally, I cannot understand why, in a civilized, compassionate and intelligent society where we do not hesitate to end the suffering of our beloved pets, we still seem incapable of granting terminally ill people, in agonizing pain and totally dependent on others, their wish to die with dignity, surrounded by loving, caring and like-minded relatives and friends.

On the subject of compassion towards sick or dying animals, the only operations I have ever performed on four-footed creatures have been fairly minor. Draining an abscess on a dog here, delivering a lamb there, treating conjunctivitis in a cat somewhere else. I may not have been as expert as a fully qualified vet but at least I was a whole lot cheaper. And I also discovered that animals on the whole make much better patients than many of us humans. My brief forays into veterinary work proved that I'd never be very good at euthanasia, which I'm sure will be reassuring for all of my patients.

Years ago, when I was working single-handed as a medical officer on the most isolated inhabited island in the world, Tristan da Cunha, one of the farmers brought his dog to me. He owned a working sheepdog called Shep who had developed uncharacteristically aggressive habits recently and had bitten one of the children quite badly. It was decided that, much as the farmer loved his dog, he would reluctantly have to put Shep down. Seeing tears in the poor man's eyes at the prospect of brutally killing his dog with a bolt through the brain from a mean-looking device called a 'humane killer', I offered him and his dog what I thought would be a more pleasant alternative. Ketamine. The animal anaesthetic. As a slow but not unpleasant lethal injection. The dog's owner jumped at the chance.

'Thank you, doctor. Thank you,' he said. 'I just couldn't bring myself to use that horrible humane killer on Shep.'

After carefully reading the pharmaceutical literature which accompanied the vials of ketamine in the box, I calculated the dose needed for normal anaesthesia and multiplied it by twenty. That should kill anything, I thought. But in a nice way. If there is such a thing. I gently administered the jab as Shep's owner patted and stroked him. Then, as the dog gradually relaxed to the floor and fell unconscious with his tongue hanging out and drooling, the two of us sat on a low stone wall nearby and talked of Shep's glory days as we watched the sun slowly set over the calm Atlantic horizon. As a spiritual place to preside over the passing of a much-loved animal, it could hardly have been better. As euthanasia goes, this wasn't a bad effort, I thought. But a few beers later, when I was just about to go and certify the dog dead and cover him up, we heard a low growl from behind us. Then a quiet bark. Then another. And a louder one. Shep had not only come round from his massive overdose, he was softly padding over to give us a little nuzzle with his snout.

'That's incredible,' I said. 'I gave him enough ketamine to kill an elephant. What do you have to use to put a dog like Shep down?'

'The humane killer, doc,' said the farmer with a rueful smile. And off he went to fetch it.

As the only doctor on the island I was also the unofficial dentist and animal welfare officer. That is why I found myself one day surgically repairing an umbilical hernia on a pig. The locals had this creature that nobody was remotely interested in raising for slaughter because of a superstition that the hernia somehow made it unwholesome or poisonous. To be honest, I felt rather sorry for it.

114

So, since there were only about 300 people on the island and I was not exactly rushed off my feet, I offered to perform corrective surgery. Armed with large amounts of ketamine, swabs, scalpel, retractor and stitches, I marched down to the farmer's field and put the beast to sleep. So far, so good. A nice little crowd of curious children gathered round to take a look, but wandered off as soon as I started the incision. To be honest, it is not a very difficult procedure. You just push the abdominal contents back into position, and while your assistant holds them there you stitch the muscles in front of the tummy firmly back together in the midline. I deliberately used great big fat dissolvable sutures as I knew the animal would go berserk when it woke up and would quickly gain a lot of weight, thus putting further strain on the tummy muscles and threatening a recurrence. After all, pigs can eat like, well, pigs.

My first veterinary operation ever was all going nicely to plan until it started to rain. And when it rains on Tristan da Cunha, it can be a deluge. I quickened my stitching rate and the wound filled with rainwater. Then the pig started to come round and kick me. I just got finished and the wound nicely strapped up before, in one deft movement, the pig rolled over on to all fours and trotted off across the meadow as if nothing had happened. It really was what they call surgery in the field.

8

Chaperones

MODERN MEDICAL ETIQUETTE DICTATES THAT EVERY MALE doctor needing to perform an examination on a female patient must offer her a chaperone if she requires one. The extra person is there not just to protect her against any overt assault or inappropriate behaviour by the doctor, but to act as a witness of events, to generally make her feel more comfortable and possibly even to hold her hand and engage her in distracting conversation. Many doctors simply point to a printed notice on the surgery wall asking their patients to read it, but I still ask them verbally whether they would like the practice nurse or receptionist to be present during the examination and almost invariably the answer is no.

Politically incorrect and insensitive though it may sound, on the very few occasions when the offer *has* been accepted, I have always been amazed at the kind of woman actually asking for a chaperone. In my experience, it has always been the kind of woman who seems least vulnerable to unwanted attention. Stern, tough, unapproachable and physically unattractive to boot. But what do I know? All I can tell you is that in over thirty years of medical practice, no one has ever made a complaint against me. In these litigious times when frivolous and often malicious complaints are sometimes made by patients with covert psychological issues, that is not only reassuring but statistically unlikely. Perhaps I shouldn't speak too soon, and certainly not without touching a forest of wood (working in TV does attract some weirdos), but I like to think I can pick up on any strange vibes I get from patients at a very early stage. Whenever I have had any niggling suspicions it has always been me who has summoned the chaperone rather than the patient.

This is because the doctor too needs protection. If a male patient comes on to a female doctor, it can create a tricky and very threatening situation. A female patient, perhaps unloved, neglected or even beaten by her partner, may develop a fixation with a male doctor she perceives as nice, attentive and caring and may deliberately dress provocatively when she attends for the examination or make suggestive remarks as he tries his best to remain objective. Wishful thinking on the medic's part, you might assume. But you would be surprised. These awkward and career-threatening situations are by no means common – I can only think of a handful of such instances in my own experience – but they can be scary. The General Medical Council and Medical Defence Union devote a fair amount of energy to warning their members of the pitfalls and suggesting how to avoid them. They also spend a lot of money and time in the High Court defending their members.

One of the problems is that lay people can easily misunderstand the nature and purpose of the examination. If a doctor enquires about a woman's sex life, it is not because he wants to pry into her personal sexual proclivities. It is because he wants to know if her libido has disappeared as part of a general backdrop of depression. If a doctor asks a woman about vaginal dryness when all she has come in to talk about are hot flushes and night sweats, it is not because he's making a clumsy pass, as some women might interpret it, but because all three symptoms are powerful indicators of the menopause.

In one well-documented legal case, a young male doctor was accused of making inappropriate advances to a female patient who had attended for a visual complaint. It turned out all he had done was to examine the back of her eye with an ophthalmoscope, looking carefully and thoroughly for any signs of optic neuritis, a typical feature of multiple sclerosis. When any doctor does this, he or she needs to get very close indeed to the patient's eye in order to look at the retina through the magnifying lens in the viewing instrument. It is no different from the very same procedure performed by an optician. Doctors often steady themselves by placing one hand on the patient's shoulder and it was this innocent manoeuvre, together with the close proximity of his mouth against her ear, which she interpreted as deep breathing, that encouraged Mrs A to believe the doctor was harbouring evil intentions.

In some cases, a woman might misinterpret a breast examination as unusual or unnecessary. This would be reasonable if she had made the appointment for treatment of a sore throat. But if she had come in for her first oral contraceptive pill prescription, or with unexplained stabbing chest pain, it might be justified. The key to avoiding such misunderstandings is, of course, for doctors to explain what it is they are doing and why. And to do this before they start the procedure. And to wait for the woman to consent to it. In many cases where complaints are brought against doctors, the problem has arisen because they have failed to do this.

In genuine cases where doctors have been guilty of gross professional misconduct, the evidence is usually overwhelming. Often it takes several women to come forward reluctantly over a period of time to corroborate the appalling experiences of others before a case reaches the courts and they can finally confront the shame, disgust and revulsion that their doctor has made them feel. Doctors are figures of authority and power, and when they abuse their position it is only right that they are heavily punished and struck off the medical register for good. Equally, women who falsely accuse male doctors of malpractice should be suitably reprimanded. The damage they can do to these doctors' careers, reputations and personal lives can be devastating and lifelong. This is why chaperones are now so often necessary and why problems can arise for either party if they are not offered.

Unfortunately, it is not always possible to provide a chaperone and that's when the real trouble starts. On a house call. With the last remaining patient of the day when the doctor is running late and all the ancillary staff have gone home. In these situations, where is the doctor's chaperone when he or she most needs one? And what about me, you're probably thinking. Didn't I ever need a chaperone in thirty years of medical practice? I did, but only on a couple of memorable occasions.

On the first, I was still training as a medical student and in the middle of a twelve-week stint in gynaecology. Dr David Knowles was an eminent gynaecologist and teacher who worked for the National Health Service at the Royal Free Hospital and had a little private practice in Harley Street on the side. As a consultant who was fluent in French, he was at one time also retained by the French Embassy in London to administer to the needs of any French female expatriates requiring the services of a gynaecologist. When he asked us students one day if any of us spoke French and would like to accompany him to his French clinic, I found myself volunteering.

There I was an hour or two later sitting in the plush consulting room of Dr Knowles's private clinic, eavesdropping on a number of young and rather attractive women as they described their medical concerns in their own charming and rather poetic language. I would have been more than happy just to sit there passively listening to Dr Knowles's gentle history-taking and expert advice and to learn from the patients' facial expressions and body language how they responded to his warm and well-practised bedside manner. Unfortunately he had other ideas.

The next patient – I'll call her Dominique – who I thought was particularly beautiful, had married relatively recently and had been coming to see Dr Knowles regularly for vaginal dilatations. She apparently suffered from vaginismus, he informed me, a not uncommon condition where the muscles surrounding the vagina go into powerful and intense spasm and make any attempt at sexual penetration impossible. The cause is psychological, often the result of sexual abuse as a child, an irrational fear of unwanted pregnancy or sexually transmitted infections, and sometimes even just an ingrained belief that all sex is sordid or dirty. Dominique had regular two-monthly appointments when she would come in, undergo her treatment and then, buoyed up with re-assurance that her vagina could comfortably and painlessly accommodate a Hegar size 9 steel dilator with the circumference of a moderate-size cucumber, go home and make love to her husband. It was a relatively straightforward procedure, Dr Knowles assured me, and while I protested that I had never performed it before, he insisted that it was well within my capabilities and that his nurse would competently assist me anyway.

A few minutes later I was standing in my long white coat next to the lovely Dominique, who was lying on the examination couch, naked apart from a flimsy white sheet covering the upper half of her lithe body. Marian, the nurse, was standing at the foot of the couch with the equipment trolley. On it was the vaginal speculum nicely pre-warmed to body temperature, the lubricating jelly piled high like a transparent walnut whip. The numerous Hegar dilators graded in size from 1 to 10 were beautifully aligned and ready for action. I snapped on the rubber gloves and checked with Dominique in the best French I could muster that she understood what we were going to do.

'*C'est toujours la même chose, non?*' she whispered demurely before nodding and turning her face away.

With some trepidation I began the procedure. Strangely, as I introduced the first torpedo-shaped silver dilator I thought my patient had taken an almost imperceptible but protracted breath. Or was I mistaken? The next, slightly wider instrument was met by a definite turning of the head to either side. The third with a low moan. The fourth prompted a slight arching of the back and the fifth a parting of the lips and some whispered words in French I couldn't quite grasp. Feeling awkward now and embarrassed despite the presence of the nurse, I hesitated to continue as it was increasingly clear that Dominique was becoming somewhat turned on. I could almost see the scandal of the court case about to be brought against me for inappropriate behaviour. The tragedy was I wasn't even qualified yet. But then Marian leaned forward and murmured in my ear.

'Don't worry,' she said matter-of-factly, 'Dominique reacts in just the same way to Dr Knowles. Just carry on.'

So I did, and incredibly Dominique endured and enjoyed the second half of the treatment in equal measure and then surprised me by expressing her gratitude and satisfaction afterwards. In retrospect it is impossible to know if having the chaperone would have avoided an accusation or not. You cannot tell what is going on in a patient's mind at any given time. Certainly not when she reacts like Dominique had done, in a bizarre and unexpected fashion. Suffice to say, both Dr Knowles and I were more than grateful the chaperone *had* been there. Without her, the situation would have been a medico-legal nightmare.

Sometimes, however, a doctor does not have the luxury of a chaperone on hand. On house calls, for instance. The second occasion on which I could really have done with a witness was when a problem occurred after I had been working as a principal in general practice for several years. I had been asked to go out and see one of my GP partner's patients who thought she had a kidney infection. A thirty-year-old teacher, she told our receptionist she had a fever and backache and was needing to use the toilet more frequently. When I got to her house six or seven miles away out in the country, I rang the doorbell and stepped inside the hall as she put her head round the door to let me in. To my great surprise, as I turned round to talk to her I saw she was completely and utterly naked. No nightdress. No towelling wrap. No dressing gown. Nothing. Not a stitch. This, I knew from years of GP experience and hundreds of house calls on all sorts of people with all types of medical complaints, was unusual. Very, very unusual. Bizarre, even. It felt like a trap.

'I'm upstairs in bed, doctor,' she said and led the way up

a short flight of stairs to the first floor, leaving nothing to the imagination. As I followed, I was thinking whether or not this was a good idea and preparing for a rapid exit should it become necessary. But what could I do? There was no prospect of a chaperone: there was no one else in the house. No neighbour or milkman on his rounds in sight. If she was really unwell, on the other hand, abandoning her would be a dereliction of my medical duty. What reason would I give? After all, she had not actually made any suggestive signal apart from waltzing around the house starkers. I wasn't going to call in reinforcements, I decided, and waste more time. I was going to go for it.

She reclined in her bed and described her symptoms. All typical, I was pleased to hear, of a genuine kidney infection. Glancing at her medical notes, I was also interested to see she had had a bout of kidney infection three years previously. Her temperature was 101 degrees F. She couldn't be inventing that. On bi-manual palpation her left kidney was acutely tender but there were no other focal signs of inflammation in her abdomen. Now I needed to test a urine sample.

Taking the small capped container with its citrate crystals at the bottom, she rose majestically from the bed and walked nonchalantly out of the room to the bathroom. The cheeks of her bottom, flushed rosy red with fever, wobbled slightly as she went and the goose pimples on her skin stood proudly to attention, as did her nipples. I tried not to notice, but doctors are trained to observe, and I remained stoically objective at all times.

The sample, when tested, was a massive relief. The urinalysis test strip showed large amounts of red blood cells. Good. Copious quantities of protein. Excellent. And white cells, nitrates and ketones. Fan-bloody-tastic. She was ill.

Sincerely and genuinely ill. I wasn't being accosted, set up, stitched up or exploited. She had real unequivocal pyelonephritis, a nasty deep-seated infection of the kidney which would leave her weak and exhausted for several days and required plenty of fluids, painkillers and antibiotics.

'I'll see myself out,' I said as I closed my medical bag and prepared to leave. 'But can I just ask you whether you always answer the door with no clothes on?'

'Oh,' she replied, 'I often walk around the house with nothing on. I grew up in Sweden where everyone does it. People here think I'm weird. I don't even have a nightdress.'

'It's just that certain doctors might be a little, well, taken aback by it. When you open the door like that.'

'OK,' she said. 'I didn't realize. My own doctor never says anything.'

I couldn't help smiling at that. Knowing her own doctor, I wasn't entirely surprised.

9

What's Up, Doc?

WHY ARE SOME DOCTORS QUITE SO USELESS? I RECENTLY saw a pal of mine who'd just returned from an out-patient appointment with an ENT specialist who told him there was nothing wrong. My friend had a severe pain in his right ear, a funny taste in his mouth, an unpleasantly loud distortion of hearing and a crop of painful blisters in his ear canal. Even I knew, as a humble GP who had never actually seen one of these cases, that it was Ramsay Hunt syndrome, a shingles infection of the geniculate ganglion, a small branch of the facial nerve lying deep within the petrous temple bone at the side of the head. Coupled with some slight weakness of the facial muscles on that side, otherwise known as Bell's palsy, the diagnosis was so obvious it was jumping up and biting me on the bum. I promptly gave him a prescription for the necessary anti-viral tablets and reassured him that all would come right in a week or two.

Then there was Jo, a neighbour of mine I met while out shopping in a local store, tearful and distraught because she'd just been told that her son had probably got a tumour in his clavicle (collar bone). She had taken him along to the last orthopaedic outpatient appointment of the day, and had been confronted by the specialist studying the X-rays. Elliot had fallen off his dirt bike on to his shoulder a few days previously and had had bouts of fever ever since, and pain when moving his arm. The doctor had apparently scrutinized the X-rays and the fuzzy blurred outline of the offending clavicle before glibly announcing that a tumour was very likely and that amputation of the arm might be required.

Jo, understandably, had been devastated. Not least because she was alone with her son in the clinic, totally unprepared and unsupported. All I could say was that I was surprised. It sounded to me much more like osteomyelitis, an infection of the bone caused by the recent trauma. The fevers would seem to fit better with this too. Two weeks and huge amounts of heart-searching later, I was proved right. Jo and Elliot were incredibly relieved and over the moon, but I couldn't take any satisfaction from it because it was not a difficult diagnosis and most doctors would have come to exactly the same conclusion as I had. But why had Jo been subjected to such unnecessary worry? Why mention the worst-case scenario first, as well as the consequences, when the original list of possible diagnoses was first made? And why do that when there was little or no time to explain the implications and provide counselling or other practical or psychological support? In my opinion, Jo and Elliot had endured a terrifying fortnight of completely unnecessary apprehension and worry. All because one doctor's communication skill was zero.

I was just thinking about this dreadful state of affairs one morning when GMTV's senior correspondent, Richard Gaisford, came over to me in the newsroom and asked me about his eyes. A couple of days previously he had noticed a funny kind of glitch in his vision which he had never before experienced, and apparently it wasn't clearing up. He described it as like a dark spot in his peripheral vision. He had been down to the A&E department at his local hospital and the ophthalmic surgeon on call examined the front of his eye and concluded that there was no corneal abrasion or ulcer and told him to go home and wait for an outpatient appointment for follow-up. Richard was asking me about it now because although his symptoms had not changed, he was going to find it difficult to make the appointment.

'You have to go back,' I said. 'It sounds to me that it might just be a retinal detachment and you can't neglect your eyesight. It's too important.'

To my amazement, the specialist had apparently not even looked at the back of his eyes.

'If you've got to go down to Devon for filming,' I suggested, 'and that's where you used to live, why not pop into a local optician down there? Opticians are usually incredibly thorough, and most of them these days are fully stocked with state-of-the-art equipment so they can check out your retina for you.'

A few days later, Richard phoned.

'Retinal detachment,' he said. 'You were right. The optician was really good and he knew the consultants at Portsmouth Hospital, so he wrote an instant referral letter and made a phone call and I got an appointment the very next day.'

'And?'

'Retinal detachment but not just in the right eye – there's a small one on the other side as well.'

Wow. Richard and I then chatted about the proposed

treatment and the implications, and how long he was likely to be off work. The treatment he subsequently had was extremely effective and straightforward, and although his eyesight is near perfect again, viewers will notice he now wears glasses when broadcasting. But how was the diagnosis missed in the first place? Why did a junior doctor wishing to specialize in ophthalmology not take the trouble to examine the back of Richard's eyes with an ophthalmoscope? Richard's problem could have been made very much worse and he was lucky that on this occasion the doctor's lack of thoroughness had not had serious consequences.

Not all the people I work with and who corner me in the corridor to ask about their health concerns are front-of-camera presenters like Richard, however. Darren Bramley is head of camera operations at GMTV and was waiting to have an operation to repair an umbilical hernia. It's OK, he doesn't mind me telling you. Obviously I asked him. He'd mentioned it a couple of times as we stood around the studio in the mornings, but he seemed to be waiting for ever to have the job done on the NHS. In this condition, a weakness in the abdominal muscles around the belly button causes the intestine beneath it to push outwards to form a soft and prominent bulge. It can occur at any age and is not usually painful unless complications arise. One day on the programme I had just finished talking about how important it was that parents should give their children the MMR vaccination when Darren asked me if he could have a quick word. It was another one of those 'What's up, doc?' moments. His hernia had become painful and unusually he had not been able to push the intestine back into place.

This rang alarm bells with me because, while an umbilical hernia is not dangerous in itself, there is always a slight possibility of its becoming strangulated if a loop of intestine is pinched by the abdominal muscles and has its blood supply cut off. If it is not attended to, this leads to gangrene and life-threatening peritonitis.

The trouble was, Darren was meant to be operating a studio camera and working until the end of the programme in two hours, and I was due back in my clinic in Hampshire at about the same time.

'You mind me taking a look right here?' I asked. 'You've got four other cameramen looking on and a few innocent bystanders besides.'

'I don't care,' he said. 'It's only my belly.'

We were on an ad break for the next two minutes, so lying him down on the same sofa that would be used just over an hour later by Lorraine Kelly for her show, I took a look at the hernia and felt it to see if it was tender. It was. Considerably.

'Hold on,' I said, and gently massaged the hernia around a little until it suddenly popped back into place inside his abdomen.

'Ow!' he said. 'But at least it's back in.'

'It is,' I said. 'But if you feel unwell, feverish or develop tummy pain in the next few hours, you'll have to go to A&E straight away just in case.'

Luckily, he didn't have to and a few weeks later he had a successful hernia repair on the NHS.

Darren was typical of studio crew. When they needed advice it was usually because of something dramatic. A head wound caused by a falling ceiling light or a blackout with convulsions for no apparent reason. Presenters, on the whole, tend to complain about more subtle symptoms. I mean if you break your leg, develop a chest infection or come down with measles, everyone knows about it right away. The onset is sudden and the change in the patient obvious. But many medical disorders creep up on people so insidiously that the diagnosis can be delayed for months or even years. Parkinson's disease, for example, can cause such gradual slowing down of movement and reduced facial expression that close family members fail to notice it. A distant cousin, however, visiting from overseas and seeing the patient for the first time in years might very well spot the change immediately. Dementia too can develop gradually, as can anaemia or thyroid problems. These are the more insidious and somewhat complicated conditions that presenters tend to bring to my attention.

Kate Garraway found this out personally when she started to suffer from an overactive thyroid after the birth of her baby, Darcy. Initially, she attributed her weight loss to breastfeeding. Others probably thought she was being very disciplined in losing some of her excess weight from pregnancy. But then her weight loss continued and observers began to comment that she looked *too* thin. Even GMTV's concerned viewers were calling in to mention it.

As Christmas approached she was eating more, yet still getting thinner. She became genuinely scared when, after eating a full English breakfast, a large lunch *and* dinner one day, she woke up the next morning weighing 1lb less than the day before. In addition, she felt hot all the time – which was unusual for her – and restless, with bags of extra energy. Darcy was now one year old and sleeping well but Kate herself was not. I even remember discreetly saying to Kate one morning that I did not think she should lose any more weight. Eventually, a blood test was done and doctors immediately discovered she was suffering severe thyrotoxicosis – a significant overactivity of her thyroid gland, which acts as the body's thermostat and energy regulator. Apparently she got a telephone call from the doctor the next day, while doing a photoshoot with Penny Smith where both of them were dressed as the *Ab Fab* characters. The doctor said she needed to come in for treatment straight away.

'Can't,' she said. 'I'm working today.'

'Got to,' replied the doc. 'The condition you have could seriously affect your heart unless we treat it.'

Thankfully, Kate's thyroid responded to the tablets she was prescribed. Although she's now off treatment altogether, she has to have follow-up blood tests every three to six months to keep an eye on things. I was pleased she got better so quickly because some months previously she had been even more unlucky when she suffered from a large kidney cyst that had become infected. Kidney cysts are very common and most people who have them remain blissfully unaware until an infection or a routine test for something else exposes them. I remembered she had been hospitalized briefly at the time and that the diagnosis had been delayed because she had found it difficult to register with a local GP. On that occasion, too, she had made a full and uneventful recovery and was soon back on the TV sofa entertaining the viewers, along with her debonair sidekick Andrew Castle.

Talking of whom, when a gorgeous, lithe and curvy dancing beauty like Ola Jordan asks a man to 'slide' when practising a samba, few hot-blooded males could refuse. A fit, ambitious Andrew, who was still very much in with a shout in the *Strictly Come Dancing* competition after several weeks, was certainly no exception, and I would not have expected anything else. I play squash from time to time with Andrew and it is obvious how he became England's erstwhile No. 1 tennis player. He is highly competitive and tries ruthlessly to win every single point without ever letting up, no matter how far ahead he may be. For any true sportsman, this is the ultimate form of flattery towards their opponent.

Unfortunately, in the excitement of sliding across the floor towards Ola on his bent knees while leaning back and shimmying his shoulders at the same time, Andrew suddenly felt something go in his knee. It hurt and immediately felt odd and less stable. The *Strictly* doctor and physiotherapist were called, and following an examination they became concerned that he might have torn a cartilage or ligament. If so, it was highly unlikely that Andrew could carry on in the competition, a bitter irony since his TV sofa partner, Kate, had also had to limp out of the previous series with a badly sprained ankle and foot problems. An MRI scan was hastily arranged to visualize the internal structure of Andrew's knee, and thankfully no serious damage was seen.

The main problem with any minor strain or injury in a thoroughbred sportsman is that it makes them apprehensive. They hold back a little for fear of aggravating the injury, and psychologically cannot commit to exercise with the same vigour and abandon. In turn this hesitation can put more pressure on other joints and muscles, threatening injury elsewhere, as well as interrupting the mental concentration required to perform the various routines. Andrew would never use an injury like that as an excuse but clearly it marred his further progress in the competition and he finally bowed out in the later stages. In a way, he told me, he was relieved. It was all very well being superfit, disciplined and committed but nothing had prepared him for the full-on eight hours a day, seven days a week rehearsals that were required and the punishing routine that Ola had been putting him through. Together with the 4am starts to present the TV breakfast show, the pressure was inevitably taking its toll. Bleary-eyed and exhausted one morning, he could hardly stammer his way through the words on the autocue. That particular day would be a good day to challenge him on the squash court, I thought, and suggested it.

'You'd probably wipe the floor with me today,' he said. 'I'm absolutely knackered.'

But I have never taken more than four points off him and I know what these 'win at all costs' sportsmen can be like. When they say things like that, you can guarantee it is a complete and utter bluff.

Ben Shepherd, our other anchor presenter, is probably just as fit as Andrew. In fact he must be the only person I work with who has *never* requested my medical advice and asked, 'What's up, doc?' He recently beat the pop singer Lemar in a televised celebrity boxing bout and hugely impressed football fans with his excellent display for England in a soccer match at Wembley against the Rest of the World for Soccer Aid – a charity raising thousands of pounds for Unicef.

One day Ben was getting all excited about meeting the PussyCat Dolls, who had come up to our London TV centre to perform their new hit single, 'When I Grow Up'. I had just finished a quick chat with him on the programme about heart attacks being common in the winter because of thicker blood and high blood pressure, but I could sense Ben was not really listening because he was looking forward so much to meeting the gorgeous girls. I was halfway out of the studio when in walked the lovely Nicole, Ashley, Jessica, Melody and Kimberly. Amazingly, one of them recognized me and came over to give me a kiss. So obviously I had to kiss them all. Out of the corner of my eye I caught sight of Ben. I had a big smile on my face. He looked gutted.

By contrast, our weather girls, or 'weather presenters' as we now have to call them, looked completely unfazed. During the hay fever season in 2008 millions of people were already suffering from streaming eyes, blocked noses and sneezing. Among them was our very own weather presenter, Andrea McLean, who had been bunged up for a fortnight and could hardly speak clearly enough to deliver her forecast and the pollen count.

'Isn't there anything I can take,' she asked me, 'other than these useless antihistamines, eye drops and nasal sprays? Something that actually works?'

'Have you ever considered having a cortisone injection?' I replied. So then we had a discussion about the pros and cons of corticosteroids in the treatment of seasonal rhinitis. Many GPs are reluctant to give them because of possible side effects. In my opinion, these have been vastly exaggerated by scare-mongering media stories, so that patients who once swore by cortisone injections and obtained dramatic relief now find it well nigh impossible to get them. In people who have already tried everything else and whose lives are made miserable by hay fever symptoms, a one-off injection of cortisone can have a near-miraculous effect. Almost overnight the symptoms clear up and the recipient stays symptom-free for several weeks – long enough usually to tide them over the entire hay fever season. There can be side effects, of course, I explained to Andrea, but they are extremely rare and usually, if they occur at all, very mild and short-lived. Nevertheless, I ran through them.

'Don't care,' she said. 'I want an injection.'

'Sure?' I asked.

'Sure.'

So between weather bulletins Andrea bent gracefully over our boss's desk, baring the upper outer quadrant of her perfectly contoured buttock as I readied myself to inject the full 2ml.

'Will I feel a little prick?' she asked mischievously.

'No. But I will if I hit a blood vessel so just keep still and shut up for a minute.'

After a quick slap to numb the skin, I plunged the needle in, emptied the syringe and the job was done. No pain. No blood. And, rather disappointingly, no cry of pleasure either. Most importantly, there were no more hay fever symptoms, according to my patient, after just thirty-six hours. Andrea certainly seemed happy and I don't know who had enjoyed the procedure most.

'So was I your first ever weather presenter?' she asked me coyly, with a laugh.

'Actually, no,' I replied. 'I gave the same treatment to Simon Keeling when he was presenting the weather a few years ago.' I remembered it well, I told Andrea, because he and I were both in a terrible hurry that day, and I administered his injection into his arm while we sat in my car in the building's underground car park. Unfortunately, just as I was pushing down the plunger of the syringe, along came the security guard, who did a quick double-take. Simon Keeling shooting up, he must have thought, with Dr Hilary acting like a drug dealer. I suddenly realized this was not the perfect place to be conducting my clinic. The guard, however, walked straight past the car without a backward glance. I could only suppose he must have been a firm believer in patient confidentiality.

Confidentiality is vital, of course, at all times for doctors but never so much as when we are asked to help out the mega-star celebrities who occasionally grace the TV studios and may have a little medical niggle of some kind. Recently, when Spice Girl Mel B's agent asked me if I would come to her changing room to check out her pulled leg muscle before she danced on the Lorraine Kelly show, I could not help reflecting on some of the special guests who have asked for my medical advice. Engelbert Humperdinck, for example, once asked me to check out his tonsils when he had a sore throat. I let Alan Davies, who played the detective Jonathan Creek, join the queue of regular staff one morning for an opportunistic flu jab. He was not allergic to eggs and nor was he pregnant so he got one. I had chatted to Charlton Heston and Jeffrey Archer about their fitness routines, talked Tony Curtis through his back problem and even had the rare privilege of examining Sinitta's strained hamstring. Nice work if you can get it.

I also recall taking a look at the late Dudley Moore's painful finger, which was getting in the way of his piano playing. Dudley, in fact, was one of my favourites. An international superstar and loved by everyone, he was always good-humoured and willing to please and there was never the slightest hint of aloofness or arrogance about him. On one occasion he was sitting minding his own business in the TV studio's Green Room when a little old lady who had won £2 million on the National Lottery heard me asking our lovely 'greeter', Brenda, whether I could have a bacon sarnie from the 'Luvvies' café downstairs. 'Of course,' said Brenda. 'I was just going down there now anyway.' And off she went. Turning to Dudley for some reason, the old lady then said, 'That sounds nice. Do you think you could get one for me?' She obviously hadn't a clue who Dudley Moore was. Much to everybody's astonishment, he jumped up with a big smile on his face, put on a high-pitched Cockney accent and said he would attend to it right away. And he did. He returned five minutes later with a well-buttered bacon sandwich and duly presented it to the elderly lottery winner, who gaily chomped her way through it without ever realizing who her celebrity waiter had been. The rest of us in the room were splitting our sides trying to contain ourselves.

Once when I was sitting in the make-up room, I noticed a figure pass by the door. Then whoever it was stopped, turned back and put their head around the door to say hello to me. To my amazement it was Tony Blair, then Prime Minister. Although he was always pleasant and affable to everyone whenever he came in, I was stunned to think he would take the trouble to say, 'Hi, doc, how are you?' when we had only ever exchanged a few words before in the same location. He had come in with Alastair Campbell prior to the previous election to talk about his party's manifesto and we had joked about what his blood pressure must be doing and how he and Alastair kept it normal by playing regular tennis together. I had liked Gordon Brown and William Hague when I'd met them too. Approachable. Pleasant. With time to listen. Unlike other politicians I might mention who refused to come on the GMTV sofa with me in case I spoilt their party by disagreeing vehemently about what they were trying to do with the NHS. Politicians, as it happens, rarely ask me about their personal health concerns. That is left to everyone else. All in all, I've seen singers with sore throats, athletes with torn muscles, dancers with sore legs and pianists with sore fingers. Now I'm just looking forward to the day when Dolly Parton comes in with a chest infection.

Sadly, I don't think that will ever happen and I will just have to make do with the occasional perks associated with looking after our in-house celebrities such as Tess Hurley. TV programmes often involve a long build-up before reveal-ing some kind of surprise. It might be announcing the winner of a competition, or revealing how somebody or something looks after a makeover. Tess, one of our loveliest producers, had agreed to be 'followed' during the course of her IVF treatment by the Lorraine Kelly *Today* show.

Starting in April, we had interviewed her about her relative subfertility, her treatments and all her hopes and aspirations for the future. She began her investigations and we filmed them. She started IVF and we covered it. Viewers identified with her predicament and phoned in in droves to support and encourage her and to wish her luck. Then, four months later, we set things up so that we could reveal on air, live on television, the results of her latest pregnancy test. I would be the presenter.

She sat, pale, nervous and trembling with concerned anticipation, in the director's office as I came in to announce the result with my cameraman following closely behind.

'It's positive!' I said. 'Congratulations! You're pregnant!'

Tess then screamed, jumped up, threw her arms around my neck and gave me a huge kiss. All in glorious close-up. I'll bet the viewers were thinking: hang on a minute, whose baby *is* this?

You get wonderful moments like this on live television. I suppose it is in the nature of the beast. But just as I was leaving the office one day to catch a train back to Hampshire, Emily McMahon, our head of sport at GMTV, stopped me in the corridor and asked if I could look at her neck. This was not surreal at all. In fact it was a very common and down-to-earth enquiry. She had noticed a painless swelling under the angle of her jaw about three weeks earlier, and it hadn't got any better since. I asked her if she had a GP but she hadn't registered with one since she moved down to London. She was incredibly busy with work, was still sprinting at athletics meetings for her county at the age of thirty-six, and anyway, she had heard what everyone else had heard – that it was well nigh impossible to get any GP in Central London to take you on these days.

It wasn't very satisfactory for me to examine her as I'm

not the company doctor. I'm also conscious of the fact that every time I give someone medical advice, I'm taking a clinical responsibility and, in theory at least, legally putting my head on a block. But hey, it's only a swollen lymph gland, I told myself, so I asked her the standard questions. Had she had a recent sore throat that would account for it? A slight sore throat, but nothing major. Earache? No. A toothache, inflamed gums, a scalp wound or an infected facial spot? Any of these problems could produce an infection that would then drain away along the chain of lymphatic glands which run vertically down the side of the neck. But again the answer was no. So we had a solitary, painless 2cm-square lymph gland of three weeks' duration or maybe slightly longer, she now said, with no obvious focal infection to explain it. She told me she had no other enlarged glands that she was aware of, but I asked her to especially check her armpits and groin as soon as she got home. I could not really examine her standing there in a busy corridor, and anyway it was not my role to do that. She had merely asked me for my opinion, that was all.

Nevertheless, I was now in a bit of a quandary. Rather reluctantly I gave her a private prescription for a broad spectrum antibiotic and insisted that I saw her when she had finished the course in one week's time. She was very grateful, she said, and headed off back to the edit suite while I rushed to catch my train.

If I'm honest, I have to admit that I did not do much speculating on Emily's problem or give her swollen neck gland another thought for the next seven days. A week later, Emily came over to me as I sat in the GMTV newsroom talking to some people who had won a studio tour in a charity raffle and were asking me what Lorraine Kelly was really like. It was a great excuse to break away and I

139

took Emily aside into the senior producer's empty office.

'How's the lump in the neck?' I asked hopefully.

'A bit better, I think,' she replied levelly.

I took a look, carefully palpating the hollow beneath the angle of her jaw on the affected side. Immediately, my heart sank. I did not think it was better at all. I had the distinct impression the lump was bigger. And possibly slightly firmer.

'You finished the whole course of antibiotics?' I asked.

'Yes. Finished a couple of days ago.'

'OK, Emily,' I said. 'I think the lump is still there. It's a solitary, painless, well-localized lymph node. There is no obvious explanation for it, and it hasn't responded to anti-biotics. Presumably you checked everywhere else for any lumps and lymph nodes as I suggested?'

'I checked and didn't find any.'

'Right. I'm not really very happy about your lump. I've seen plenty of people with similarly enlarged glands which, bizarrely, and for no obvious reason, gradually disappear after several weeks. Things like glandular fever, deep-seated dental abscesses and non-specific inflammation can all cause this. But if I'm honest with you – and especially since you are not yet registered with a GP and I'm not always around – I do feel you should see an ENT surgeon for a second opinion. Do you want me to arrange it?'

Emily did, and since she didn't mind travelling down to Hampshire where I knew the surgeon personally, I fixed up an urgent appointment. I should really have been half expecting the phone call I got from the surgeon a few days later, confirming Emily's diagnosis. At thirty-six, this slim, healthy and otherwise extremely fit young woman had cancer of the tonsil which had spread to the lymph glands in her neck. Shortly after, I took a phone call from Emily herself, who, as you can imagine, was devastated.

Head and neck cancer is never an easy condition to face up to or treat and I realized straight away what she was going to have to go through. But you do not get to be a county athletics champion without guts and courage and Emily had both in spades. Although off work for a few weeks, she made steady if stuttering progress and with the support of her family she soon came to terms with her cancer and, despite pain and difficulty with swallowing, endured her radiotherapy stoically. I had spoken to her oncologist about a new monoclonal antibody treatment for head and neck cancer called cetuximab, which clinical trials suggested could improve the outcome for patients when given simultaneously with radiotherapy. Currently, however, because of its cost, NICE had not yet approved it for NHS use, and Emily herself was in no position to fund the treatment. Luckily, soon after, NHS funding in Emily's case was secured and it looked as if, at least for the time being, things were starting to go Emily's way. I certainly hoped so. She was aware of a strong history of various cancers among her close relatives but her healthy lifestyle made her diagnosis particularly cruel and unfair.

Several months later, Emily was doing really well. Her treatment for head and neck cancer was completely finished, she had been back at work for some time and was once again running competitively. All her medical follow-up was good, and there was no sign whatsoever of anything untoward. While no doctor will ever actually say it, it really does seem as if she has been completely cured. When I think back to that casual encounter in the corridor at work all those months ago, I always wonder what might have happened if I'd been on holiday for a few weeks or working abroad on a special project of some kind. No doubt Emily would have seen another doctor and been treated in just the same way. But no one can ever know how significant any delay to the diagnosis may prove. It just shows how dangerous it is that so many patients find access to a GP so difficult these days. And it demonstrates just how much responsibility any doctor takes on when answering even the most apparently trivial question in an informal setting.

I was delighted and thrilled to be in a position to help Emily in the early stages and recognize the problem, and although Emily was amazingly and unnecessarily grateful, we were just lucky. In retrospect, it would have been so easy to have told her that the condition would slowly improve and not to worry, but some sixth sense and medical instinct made me take it further early on. It was the specialists who carried out the really important work and saved her life, but it was good at least to feel part of the team. The same team, incidentally, that scratches my back while I scratch theirs. The occasional complimentary theatre ticket, corporate box invite to Twickenham Rugby Football Ground or upgrade to business class on a long-haul flight to Cape Town does not grow on trees, you know . . .

10

The Oxford Union

WOW. I'D BEEN INVITED TO SPEAK AT THE OXFORD UNION. I was really flattered. It might not be the sexiest subject I had ever been asked to debate, but you don't turn down offers to stand up and talk on the same hallowed ground where once Nelson Mandela, Mother Theresa and Bill Clinton enthralled students and members of the public alike.

The motion was 'The NHS is safe only in government hands'. I was going to oppose it. Vehemently. After years of political interference and reform which in my view had almost destroyed rather than improved the NHS, I was going to argue that ministers should stop meddling and allow it to be run as a completely independent body and free from political manipulation and spin. I was planning to say that the existing arrangements led to poor decision-making, plummeting staff morale and deteriorating relationships between doctors and their patients. The pressure on politicians to win elections on the back of empty promises simply forced the NHS to operate within unmanageably brief political timescales, when what was actually needed was a long-term perspective providing people who really knew what they were doing with the power to make difficult decisions without having to worry about the political impact. That was what I intended to say, and that was what I had prepared.

Unfortunately, the other three speakers arguing against the motion with me all wanted the NHS to be privately run or partially privately run instead. But I was completely opposed to this too. I suddenly felt I should be sitting all on my own on a third independent bench, or at least, after hearing the first two speakers proposing the motion, siding with them. Having eight speakers on this rather dry subject was, as it turned out, a mistake. The opening speeches took too long, and slowly people began to doze off. This was not surprising as many students had finished their end-of-term exams that very same day. By the time I stood up, it was late and I felt like being provocative. It was time to wake up and smell the coffee.

'The NHS is one of the world's largest employers with 1.3 million staff. Its annual budget is £100 billion and it currently takes up 9 per cent of our GDP. Obviously an institution like this requires considerable organization.' So far so good, I thought. 'But this government and others before them couldn't organize a piss-up in a brewery, a knock-up in a brothel, a cock-up in an erectile dysfunction clinic or, with the possible exception of the deputy prime minister, John Prescott, a punch-up at Madison Square Garden.'

The students seemed to like this, particularly the medical analogy of the cock-up.

'It's a real privilege,' I went on, 'to be here to speak on this subject at the Oxford Union, not just because of the historical setting but because, of the eight speakers here this evening, I'm the only one who actually works in the NHS. As a practising doctor, I regularly see patients and listen to their worries, I get my hands dirty and I diagnose and administer treatments. But usually us doctors are the *last* people anyone would ever ask how best to run the health service. After all, what would *we* possibly know? For that matter, what would nurses, physios, occupational therapists and all the other dedicated health care professionals who make up the 1.3 million employees seeing 1 million patients every single day possibly be able to contribute to making the NHS run more efficiently? Politicians don't seem to think we can be trusted to spend taxpayers' money wisely. They think we should leave it to them. But I don't believe for a moment that the NHS is only safe in government hands. In fact, the way it's going, I cannot see the NHS as we now know it lasting more than another ten years.

'Conceived a few years previously, the NHS was finally born after a difficult and prolonged delivery on 5 July 1948 and it was a very, very precious baby. During the war, everyone had suffered together and the idea was that in peace everybody would benefit together also. It was to be available to everybody, equitable, of high quality, comprehensive and free at the point of delivery. It would support us from the cradle to the grave and from the womb to the tomb. Aneurin Bevan dubbed it "the greatest socialist achievement of the labour government". And I personally have been very proud to work in it for the last thirty years.

'But now,' I said, 'the NHS is sixty years of age and riddled with political cancer. The founding principles have been betrayed by successive governments which care less for the medical welfare of patients and more about winning elections on empty promises. How could we contemplate private firms taking over failing hospitals?' I asked. 'Profit-making companies paid for with public money and answerable to shareholders could only be cost-effective by providing nice, easy operations which pay well, such as varicose vein and hernia operations, while other patients were abandoned. Who would be interested in looking after the long-term chronically sick, the people with multiple sclerosis, with mental health issues, with addictions and eating disorders? Where is the profit in them? We would have to pity the elderly, anyone with cancer, premature babies and anyone seeking infertility treatment. Privately run, government-commissioned hospitals would not be interested in anyone like that. Already we have a situation where hospital managers penalize the consultants with the longest waiting lists. But what is it about those long waiting lists that managers don't understand? It's precisely *because* those consultants provide the best service and actually spend time talking to patients that everybody wants to see them. It's the consultants with the *shortest* waiting lists who should be punished. Why don't GPs refer patients to them? It's obvious, isn't it?

'We should be equally wary of Lord Darzi's vision of future general practice in polyclinics. Millions of pounds are going to be devoted to the setting up of polyclinics where twenty-five or more GPs will administer to more than fifty thousand patients, providing extended hours and extra services. But what would the difference be between a polyclinic like this and a hospital? How will an ageing population travel the twenty miles or so to get to such a polyclinic with their failing eyesight, arthritic joints and dodgy balance? They will certainly have to try, because local general practices will be shut down, their budgets slashed, their staff poached and their leases torn up.

'There is also the real worry of everyone forgetting all

about the doctor/patient relationship and continuity of care. The chances of you seeing the same doctor twice would become less than they already are. Not so long ago, the NHS could provide equal care for everyone, independent of class or status. Now we have a postcode lottery where somebody living on one side of the street can obtain a drug for cancer and somebody on the other side cannot. In one region a patient with multiple sclerosis can have a disease-modifying drug prescribed, whereas patients in other regions cannot. Some can obtain life-prolonging medications for breast, bowel and lung cancer, others cannot. In Scotland and Wales you get free prescriptions and free care for the elderly. In England we cannot.

'Not so long ago the NHS could provide comprehensive care. But now, sufferers of age-related macular degeneration, one of the commonest causes of blindness, have to go blind in one eye before they can contemplate having treatment in the other. Many special care baby units are supported almost entirely by charity rather than the state. In most areas infertility treatment is rationed.

'The relentless pursuit of achieving targets in hospitals has betrayed patients also. Some 32,000 beds have been lost in the last year on the altar of trying to achieve 100 per cent bed occupancy to satisfy government projections. But this leaves no time for the cleaning of wards because one patient is admitted as the other is discharged. Private cleaning firms win tenders on the basis that they are cheapest and then use one mop to push germs around an entire department. This is one of the reasons why we have record levels of superbugs killing hundreds of patients every month. Even the private firms that were hired to sterilize surgical instruments have succeeded in supplying broken, contaminated equipment resulting in hundreds of cancelled operations. And private hospitals commissioned to take on overspill tasks the NHS is unable to carry out have only done 50 per cent of the work they were paid to do. The continuing existence of mixed-sex wards is a national disgrace, and our care of the elderly is shameful, offering no hope, no dignity and no comfort. Little wonder death rates from clostridium difficile have increased ten times among our old age pensioners.

'It is only the dedication and tireless efforts of our staff that actually keep the NHS going. But how are *they* treated by the government? Look what happened when the government changed NHS consultants' contracts. Ministers were convinced that hospital consultants spent more time on the golf course than with their patients. They insisted they would only be paid for the work they did. Consequently, they soon discovered that consultants were already doing far more work than they were being paid for, and therefore the workload had to decrease while the expenditure stayed the same. What a ridiculous political own goal. The government promised that every new mother in labour would have her own individual midwife. The Royal College of Midwives soon realized this was a complete joke. Midwives are currently having to run from one room to another attending three women in labour at the same time. Babies' lives have been put at risk because of a cash-strapped NHS cutting jobs when demand for extra skills is soaring. Ninety per cent of newly qualified midwives are without a job, as are health visitors, physiotherapists, occupational therapists and district nurses. Governments cannot afford the £2.50 daily to provide drugs for hundreds of thousands of patients with Alzheimer's disease, while hospital managers are running around taking out one in three light bulbs in hospital corridors to save money.

'The government is shutting down many of the local hospital emergency and maternity units in order to merge them with regional superhospitals ten or twenty miles away. But if money is a problem, and most people realize it will always be limited, why are we wasting it? Why have successive governments wasted millions on a recruitment campaign for nurses when qualified nurses cannot find posts to apply for, and at a time when health visitors are being replaced by inadequately trained nursery nurses? Why do they waste millions on national surveys asking what patients want in their NHS when it is so manifestly obvious? Why do they allow the loss of £268 million spent on health tourism, when people who have no right whatsoever to NHS treatment come and leech off British taxpayers who deserve better treatment themselves? Why have successive governments appointed more managers to oversee the sacking of front-line clinical staff, to the extent that there are now more administrative staff in the NHS than doctors and nurses? Why have they allowed a situation where an incredible 10 per cent of the entire NHS budget is spent on litigation to defend the service against complaints that have been made due to mistakes caused by inadequate management? Even worse, up to £20 billion has been wasted on a disastrous national programme for IT which no one wanted, does not work and remains years behind schedule. I was even personally threatened with litigation for stating my opinions about this by a very aggressive PR company which the government was presumably paying handsomely to defend it.

'Instead, the government choose the soft targets. They charge people for parking their car in hospital grounds so that relatives of the terminally ill and of children having chemotherapy for leukaemia can be financially fleeced at an incredibly emotional time. I despair. Politicians used to say that doctors were arrogant. They used to say that the only difference between a doctor and God was that God didn't think he was a doctor. But today, it seems all that arrogance has rubbed off on politicians instead.'

I finished my talk at the Oxford Union by stating that we should not allow government to go on destroying our wonderful NHS in this way, and that it will only be safe if taken *out* of government hands. Then I appealed for them to vote *against* the motion. But if I thought I'd done a reasonable job, it was nowhere near as brilliant and entertaining as Dr Richard Smith's contribution which followed. Better known as the former editor of the *British Medical Journal* and now working for the largest health care company in the US, the United Health Group, he assessed the atmosphere in the hall, noted the late hour and readjusted his speech accordingly. He stood up and performed an impromptu and virtuoso little dance in front of us all, while giving an inspired and highly amusing rendition of the famous cockney ditty 'The Winkle Song' at the same time. Oxford had never seen anything like it and it brought the house down.

Soon after, the speakers and students repaired to the union bar to discuss medical politics, end-of-term exams and more salacious media matters. Former Atomic Kitten singer Kerry Katona had shocked viewers a few days before when she appeared on *This Morning* with Fern Britton and Phillip Schofield badly slurring her words but indignantly denying she had been drinking. The reality TV star who had previously battled drug addiction rambled so incoherently that viewers were immediately phoning up to express their concern.

Phillip asked, 'You don't seem right to me. You've got

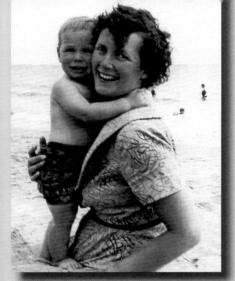

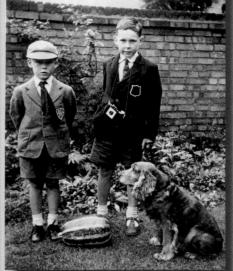

Above left: Having a cuddle with mum Noreen, aka 'Noggy', on the beach at Bournemouth aged eighteen months.

Above right: Little goody two shoes – with my older brother Nick in the garden outside my dad's surgery in Chiswick.

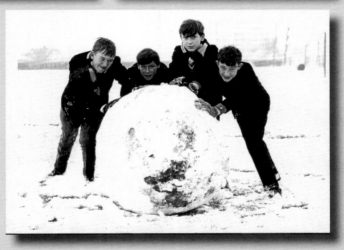

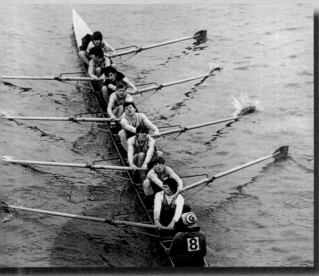

Above: Me (*second left*) with schoolmates Mel Smith, Tom Sunderland and Gwyn Hopkins. Tom, one of my best friends, tragically died of leukaemia shortly after this photo was taken. I cried a lot and began to think of a career in medicine.

Left: Stroking the Latymer School First Eight in the head-of-the-river race. I rowed with a temperature of 38.5 degrees that day. Stupid really.

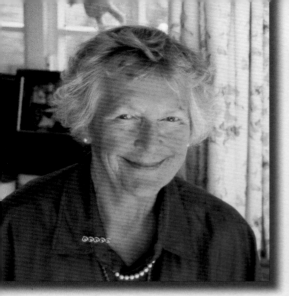

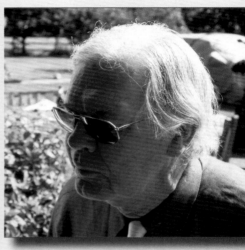

My fantastic mum, Noggy, loved by all. Especially me.

My inspirational GP dad, Evan. A great and popular doctor who treated every patient as he would wish to be treated himself.

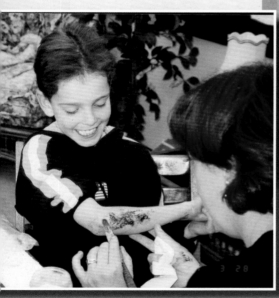

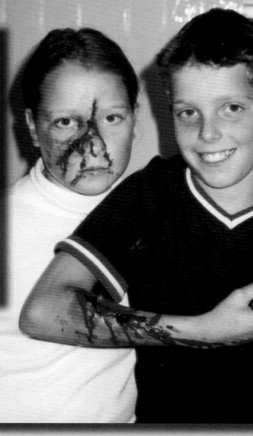

Above: My son Ru looks on gleefully as the make-up girl from *Casualty* artificially creates a hideous laceration.

Right: And my daughter, Sammy, joins in with a nasty machete wound across her nose.

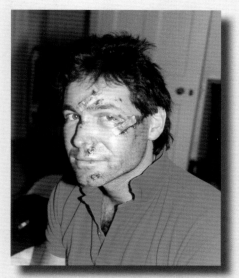

Recovering from concussion and two dozen stitches in my face after a push-bike accident.

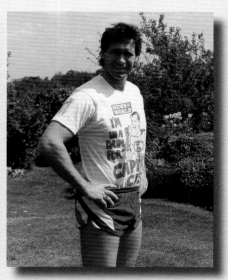

Training for the New York marathon in 1993. In some countries these shorts are actually illegal!

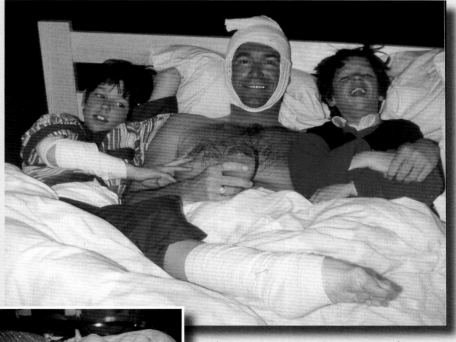

Above: Recuperating after Sebastian (*on my left*) embedded his skis in the top of my head. Tristan is wrapped in the rest of the bandages.

Left: One of the twins in special care, struggling to stay alive after being born twelve weeks early.

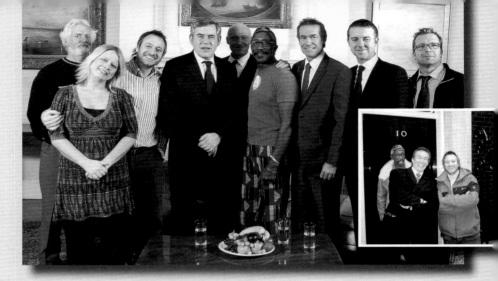

Above: At Number 10 with Prime Minister Gordon Brown and some of the GMTV team, all trying to get the nation fitter.
© GDAVIESPHOTO.COM

Above inset: Trevor Le Jeune and me outside Number 10 Downing Street with Derek Evans, aka Mr Motivator, the man tipped to be the next prime minister, just behind us.
COURTESY TREVOR LE JEUNE

Left: Tagging the ear of a rare white rhino at Shamwari in South Africa.

Below: Fiona Phillips and me with a little Zulu warrior at Shamwari, where we released two lions into the wild for the Born Free Foundation.

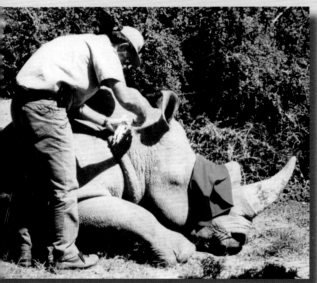

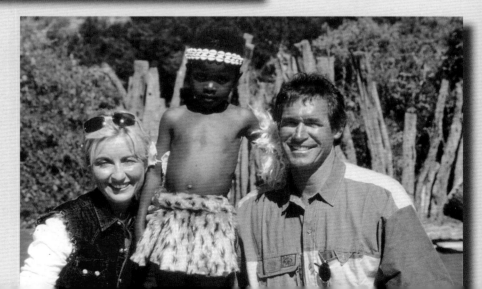

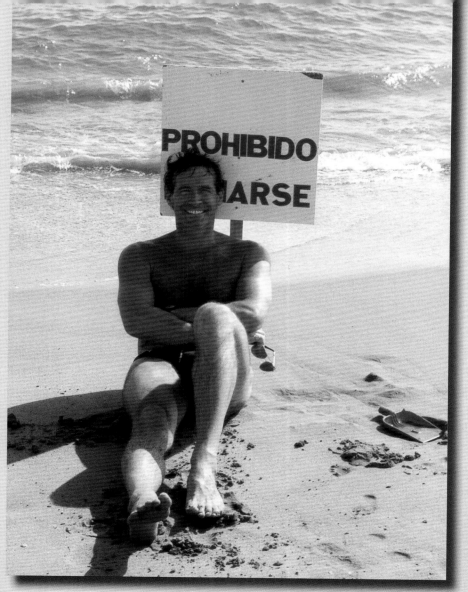

Above: *Fun in the Sun* was one of GMTV's most popular programmes. But there were limits, as you can see.

Right: Relaxing in the soothing volcanic spa waters of the famous Blue Lagoon in Iceland.

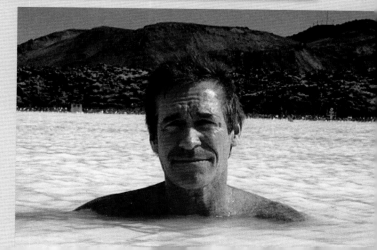

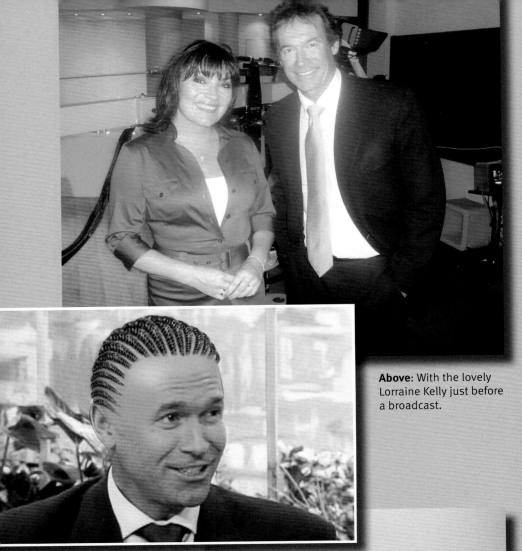

Above: With the lovely Lorraine Kelly just before a broadcast.

Above: A chat about trichology brings out the best in the computer graphics department.

Right: Newsreader Penny Smith (32) at one of her more normal moments.

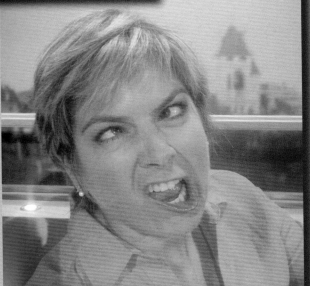

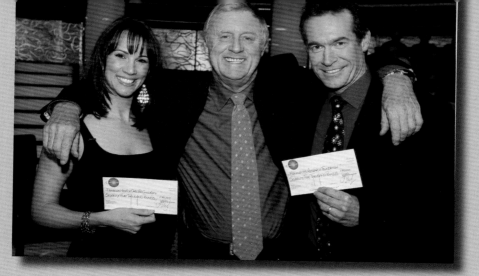

Above: Chris Tarrant presents Andrea McLean and me with cheques totalling £250,000 for charity on *Celebrity Millionaire*.

Right: Chris Tarrant tries out a very attractive CPAP mask as a cure for snoring.

Below: Morning surgery with the gorgeous Girls Aloud. Nice work if you can get it.

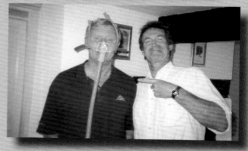

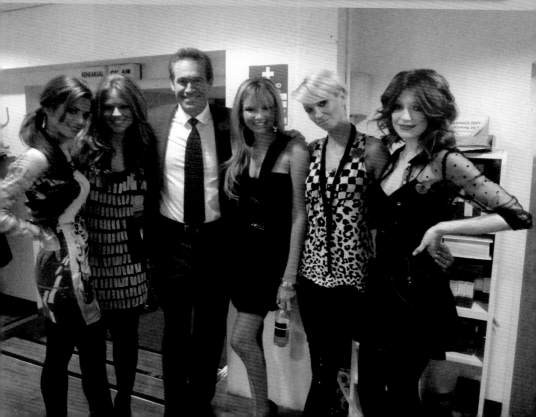

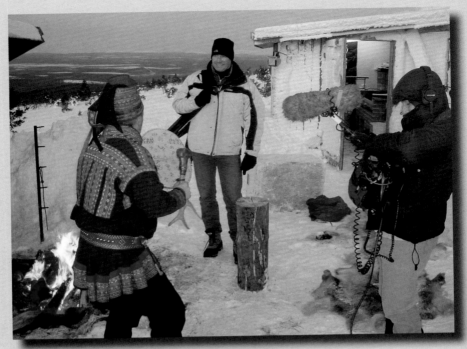

Above: Freezing cold at minus 15 degrees Centigrade for the traditional Reindeer Ceremony in the Arctic Circle. So why all the fuss about Lap Dancers?

Below: Joining the wonderful Northern Lights Charity on their annual trip to take children with life-limiting illnesses to meet the real Santa in Lapland.

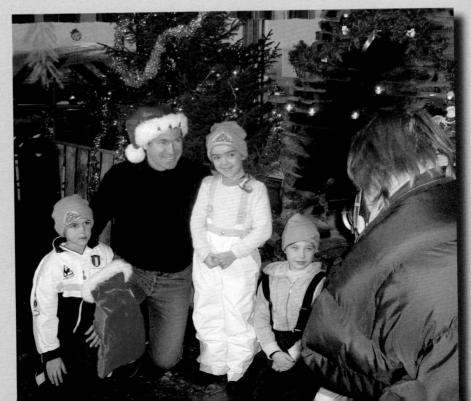

your body sorted [they had been discussing the recent cosmetic surgery she had had on her breasts together with some liposuction] but your speech is a bit slurred. How are you feeling?'

Kerry seemed surprised at this, glanced off camera and said, 'Is it? That's probably because I'm on medication at night-time, which I took at half past eleven last night. I was on a TV show last night. I wasn't talking like this yesterday, probably because it's early in the morning. I've got it with me – it's 150mg of chlorpromazine.' Then she added, with more insight than she could possibly have imagined, 'Now this is going to be made into a huge, big publicity thing. I'm absolutely fine, all it is is my medication. I swear to God, I'm absolutely fine.'

Within minutes of the interview, such was the sensation it caused, it could be viewed by millions on YouTube and *This Morning*'s own website. Radio shows were full of it for the rest of the day, with comments from her publicist, Max Clifford, who had apparently not known anything about the interview in advance, and the following day's newspaper headlines drew further attention to Kerry's troubles. Everybody seemed to have an opinion on the subject so it was almost inevitable that I would be asked for a medical one on breakfast TV. I was fully aware of earlier reports about Kerry's previous drug addiction and troubled social life, much of which she had been very open about in numerous articles and broadcasts. But this was genuine car-crash TV and everyone could see for themselves what was happening live on air.

'I have never seen Kerry as a patient. I am not her doctor. I cannot diagnose her and she says she hasn't been drinking. We have to respect that,' I said when interviewed the next day. I knew this would keep the lawyers happy – and nobody likes to be sued. Sometimes, in these speculative situations, however, you would look professionally foolish if you did not state the most obvious explanation, but you have to phrase it in a way which is not libellous but allows anyone with an iota of intelligence to read clearly between the lines.

'But if somebody exhibiting these symptoms and this kind of behaviour came into my surgery, I would certainly be concerned about them and want to find out what medication they were taking and for what condition. A hundred and fifty milligrams of chlorpromazine is a very big dose, a maintenance dose used for conditions like schizophrenia and bipolar disorder. But it shouldn't be causing severe disabling side effects the following day if the dose is correct. I'd have to assume a person who showed such side effects was drinking, or that the medication was interacting with some other medication or drug.'

Ben Shepherd then asked me about the possible side effects of chlorpromazine, reading out some of the emails our viewers had sent in.

'Dry mouth, abnormal movements, agitation, blurred vision, drowsiness – are these all possible consequences of taking it?' he asked.

'Yes,' I said. 'And there are many other possible explanations for why someone might appear intoxicated. Low blood sugar in diabetics, for example.' Hypoglycaemia can easily lead to confusion, strange behaviour, staggering and slurred speech and many a diabetic has been accused of being drunk because of it. 'Head injury, brain abscess, acute confused states due to fever . . . There are lots of reasons why somebody could appear drunk. Kerry says she had not been drinking so maybe there was another, innocent explanation.'

152

It is always difficult speculating on the mental and physical health of people in the public eye, yet it is precisely *because* these people are in the public eye and talk about themselves so readily that, when problems arise, everybody wants to know what is going on. In fact, any discussion on the subject becomes something all the rest of us can learn from. There are the gawpers, the rubber-neckers, the cynics and the simply curious, for sure. But there are equal numbers of people who are genuinely sympathetic and supportive and who draw strength and encouragement from other people's woes because they make their own problems and difficulties that bit more normal and acceptable.

Why though, I couldn't help thinking, is anybody on such a high dose of powerful sedative medication, who has had such a turbulent social life and dabbled with drug abuse, putting themselves forward for live TV interviews? Why would they want to brag about the £15,000 worth of cosmetic surgery they have just had to change the size of their breasts, and how could qualified surgeons ethically justify undertaking such an operation in someone so obviously fragile? Don't celebrities pay minders and PR agencies to guard them? Don't they have partners and other loved ones to protect them? Max Clifford, I know, is incredibly protective and responsible towards all his clients. Whenever I have met him, I have always been impressed by his professionalism and modesty. But it was reported that he didn't know anything about this interview and if he had, I am sure he wouldn't have allowed it to take place.

Shortly after this debacle, it was reported that Max and Kerry had parted company. But others knew about the interview, and maybe they should look at their own motives. MTV executives were allegedly in the studio eager to gain promotion in any way possible for their weekend

programme *Whole Again*, featuring Kerry, in a few days'
time. You have to wonder if there really is such a thing as
bad publicity. Not as far as they are concerned, maybe.
Either way, my own view is that vulnerable people who have
struggled to overcome psychological problems, and whose
recovery is still fresh and new, should be steered well away
from the limelight and protected from themselves. The
bright media spotlight in Britain is not the place to be if
mental and physical rehabilitation is required, and if a quiet
and peaceful life is what you need most.

Out-of-control celebrities are not the only ones drinking
themselves into oblivion. Britain's binge-drinking culture is
worse than ever, with one in three men and one in five
women drinking more than the recommended safe amounts.
As the Christmas party season approached, police were
bracing themselves for yet another month of hell when
violence and mayhem would inevitably erupt on our streets
and fill NHS A&E units with the victims of fighting, alcohol
intoxication and serious road traffic accidents.

To highlight the problem, I was sent up to Newcastle –
one of the UK's binge-drinking capitals – to film on the
streets and in the pubs and bars and discover just how bad
the situation had become. It certainly would not be an easy
shoot – people who are drunk are often disorderly and love
nothing more than to deliberately ambush any cameraman
or presenter's attempts to go about their work. To make
matters worse, the TV company had sent me up there with
a producer I shall call M, someone I hadn't worked with
before but who I quickly discovered had Tourette's
syndrome. Now don't get me wrong. I have nothing against
people with Tourette's syndrome. It is a highly mis-
understood condition which many people, through

ignorance, find funny because of the involuntary and frequent expletives that emerge from the mouths of sufferers as a means of relieving stress. It is like a nervous tic – where a rude utterance such as the f-word is dropped into normal conversation just as other people say 'um', 'er', 'like' or 'you know'. But it is totally beyond their voluntary control and, without intelligence, hard work and great attitude, victims can easily become marginalized and isolated from the rest of society. Just getting a job and forming normal relationships can be an uphill battle.

The evening started badly as M and I queued to get through airport security. Surrounded by a mass of excited schoolchildren, it soon became obvious that M had come to terms with his Tourette's long ago and, if anything, had overcompensated for it with no lack of self-confidence and nonchalance. As he loudly told me what we were to film when we arrived in Newcastle, the children's teachers were shocked at the language pouring from his mouth.

'We've got to get into some fucking bars and fuck, fuck, ask the girls particularly why they fuck, fuck, fucking drink before they even leave the fucking house, you know.'

'M,' I said, 'keep it down, mate. Tell me later.'

But M was having none of it. He seemed oblivious to the reaction he was causing. Worse still, the headteacher had clocked me as the doctor off the TV and was clearly wondering what kind of company I kept. He was giving me a look as if to say that that nice Dr Hilary seems to be going on holiday with a strange, dishevelled young man who acts as if he's off his face on drugs. Luckily, the flight was only a quick one-hour shuttle up to the North East, and passed uneventfully as M was distracted with a couple of beers, which helped to calm down his Tourette's.

Then we hit the town centre and set up the camera. Girls

as young as twelve or thirteen in temperatures of minus 2 degrees C were coming along the street wearing almost nothing and trying their best to walk properly in five-inch killer heels. Their miniskirts were no wider than belts and their plunging necklines almost reached their middle. Unfortunately, lack of exercise, obesity and excess drinking allow fat to bulge out in unattractive places and the overall impression created by the skimpy fashions was not that great. Several groups of them were holding each other up because they had deliberately had a bottle of wine each before leaving home because it was cheaper to become intoxicated that way than buying drinks out. They had come out now because it was 'happy hour' and for the next sixty minutes they could get a lot of drinks down their necks for just half the price. After that, the blokes would buy the drinks in return for a bit of flirting made all the easier by the increasing levels of inebriation. As I walked past a row of waiting taxis, the signs on every one clearly stated that a £50 fine applied to anyone who vomited in the back of a cab. Obviously it was a common occurrence.

My attention was suddenly drawn to a fracas going on behind. Something was kicking off already. When I turned round to take a look I saw M arguing with a burly and very unamused bouncer because they wouldn't let him in to film binge drinking on their premises.

'It's fuck, fuck, fucking TV we want to do in here,' he was saying, his arms gesticulating madly. 'We just fuck, fuck, fuck want to fucking show what goes on when people fuck, fuck, fucking binge, you know . . . We'll just be fuck, what, fuck, fucking ten minutes . . . That, fuck, OK?'

The bouncer stared silently back. Nutter, he was thinking. Pissed nutter at that. Pissed, rude nutter who needed escorting well away from that drinking joint. So I stepped in.

'He's with me,' I said. 'It's OK, that's M, he's my producer.'
Fortunately the bouncer had seen my face on breakfast telly
and began to relax.

'What's up, doc?' he said. 'What's going down?'

So I explained what we were trying to do and rather
reluctantly he let us in on the proviso that we didn't identify
the premises. Inside, groups of loud, uncoordinated girls
boasted that they could drink their boyfriends under the
table any time. They could not name any serious consequences of excess drinking, and they were not in the
slightest bit concerned about missing work the next morning because of a hangover.

'It's not so bad if you're sick,' said one helpfully.

'What's Lorraine Kelly like?' said another, losing the
thread already. 'I really fancy Ben Shepherd. He's fit.'

Over-made-up pole dancers of about seventeen cavorted
clumsily around their sticks as spotty blokes with glazed
eyes ogled them and simultaneously sipped their pints. It
was a good night out, it really was. Outside in the street
again, increasing numbers of young people were sitting with
their head in their hands, bent over the contents of their
stomach spattered between their feet.

'That's fuck, fuck, fucking disgusting,' said M, relieving a
bit more of the stress he was feeling.

Incredibly, this was not even a Saturday night in
Newcastle. It was Thursday. What is clear is that binge
drinking is no longer a once-a-month or twice-a-year
extravaganza to celebrate something special. It is a regular,
maybe two or three times a week activity for many people,
with no reason or excuse necessary other than that getting
as drunk as a skunk helps them escape the reality of their
lives. They can do this because alcohol is so affordable.
Special loss-leader deals in supermarkets, happy hours in the

pubs and clubs and 'girls drink for free' promotions have made it so. Alcohol is also more palatable for younger people these days, with sweet-flavoured drinks like Alcopops outselling bitter and spritzers.

We carried on filming in the clubs and in the town centre until around 2am and then retired to the satellite truck to send the footage back to London to be edited for the next morning's programme. I hoped it would raise awareness of the worrying epidemic of teenage binge drinking in every major town centre in the UK. With a few last f-words, M said goodnight to me and the camera crew and I turned in for a few hours' sleep. Lying in bed in my hotel room, I could not help reflecting on what I had seen. I hoped that my comments during my outside broadcast from a deserted but litter-strewn Newcastle town centre the next morning would highlight the very real dangers and consequences of bingeing on alcohol.

Forty per cent of all admissions to casualty departments are now alcohol-related. Between midnight and 5am this rises to 70 per cent. There are 22,000 premature deaths caused by alcohol each year and the NHS spends £2.7 billion putting people back together from the terrible effects of excess booze, a figure which does not even include the huge additional cost of dealing with alcohol-related crime and social problems. A report from the Prime Minister's own strategy unit confirms that 1.3 million children are affected by parents with drinking problems and that a very high proportion of them will go on to copy that behaviour and become alcoholics themselves. All in all, it is a very bleak picture indeed.

The government's chief medical officer recently stated that heavy drinking in young people is leading to an alarming rise in cases of cirrhosis of the liver. Cirrhosis –

permanent scarring and shrinkage of the liver – has seen an eight-fold increase in deaths among men and a seven-fold increase among women. It now kills 1,600 women a year compared to just 1,200 seven years ago – more lives than are lost as a result of cervical cancer. But it is not just the liver that is poisoned by too much alcohol. Almost every organ in the human body is harmed by ethanol – a chemical toxin – including the brain and the nervous system. Often the effects are irreversible.

Research from the Portman Group, the industry's own advisory body, shows that up to 1 million young men and women deliberately drink to get drunk. It seems they see sensible drinking and having a good time as mutually exclusive pursuits. In the Queen's Speech of November 2008 the Home Secretary, Jacqui Smith, announced sweeping new laws to crack down on public drunkenness. Fines of £2,500 for yobs caught boozing in the street and £500 penalties for under-eighteens caught with alcohol, who will also have their drink confiscated by the police. An end to cut-price promotions, all-you-can-drink and women-drink-free offers too. Shops losing their licences the second time they are caught selling booze to under-eighteens. Given enough police resources and stringent enforcement these measures could certainly help, but the real challenge is surely to make drunkenness and alcohol intoxication as socially unacceptable as drunk driving or physical abuse. So what is to be done? How can this socially damaging slippery slope be cleaned up?

In the ninety seconds of remaining air time the next morning I tried to summarize a few steps that might help. Simply making alcohol more expensive isn't the answer. People would find a way round it or just make their own. But if happy hours and two-for-one deals in supermarkets were stopped it would discourage the rapid consumption of large volumes of alcohol. We need better education in schools too. If we accept that sex education and information about the dangers of drugs are important, surely a campaign to raise awareness of the hazards of probably the most abused drug of all – alcohol – has to be important too? We need role models to talk to kids about the advantages of drinking alcohol in moderation – to enjoy its pleasant benefits but avoid its extremely unpleasant consequences when consumed in excess. We need to show that real drunkenness is not pretty. And for young people particularly – who may not care about health consequences thirty years from now – we need to show how their appearance can suffer in the short term as a result of obesity, bad skin and faster ageing. We need to appeal to their vanity. Parents need to lead by example too, while young recovered alcoholics with or without cirrhosis need to go into schools and talk to their peer group about their dreadful experiences caused by the bottle. Finally, more young people need support as they search for a responsible direction in life and the motivation and inspiration to achieve something valuable for themselves and others. Society needs to help them find more to life than this round-the-clock psychological and physical dependence on alcohol.

The following day I was invited on to *The Alan Titchmarsh Show* to debate the subject of the current GP contract with columnist Carole Malone. I like and admire Carole, not least because of her entertaining and indignant attacks on Anne Diamond, who had been so economical with the truth about her own gastric band surgery despite having taken part in *Celebrity Fit Club*, the same TV weight-loss programme as Carole was on herself. Carole, who had lost a considerable amount of weight the hard way, looked healthy and slim when I saw her, and we happily chatted away back-stage before we came on. We both knew we were there to be combative as well as entertaining, and we duly took our places in front of a full and attentive audience.

'Hilary, doctors are apparently earning up to £250,000 a year on the NHS despite doing less work. That can't be right, can it?' began Alan.

'No. And it isn't,' I said. 'I think one solitary doctor in the whole of the NHS has been quoted as having earned that amount of money gross, but he was doing the job of two doctors, and after expenses his salary was considerably less than that. The average GP earns around £60,000 a year.'

'Nevertheless, it does seem a lot of money when many patients don't seem to be able to get medical help out of hours when they most need it.'

'I couldn't agree more, Alan. The new contract allowed doctors to opt out of twenty-four-hour cover for their patients without the government making any proper or tested provision for emergency care out of hours. It was bad for patients, bad for medicine and short-sighted of doctors, who didn't seem to realize they would lose all that good will built up over the last sixty years.'

Carole jumped in at this moment and told a sad and heartfelt tale about her own mother, who had struggled with a chronic and debilitating illness with very little practical help, understanding or support from her doctors. I agreed that this was unacceptable, and also said it was a shame that patients and their relatives are having to fight so hard for a decent basic level of medical care.

'It's obscene what you doctors earn,' she continued, and suggested that the GP contract be torn up forthwith.

'It is an obscene amount,' I agreed, before adding, much

to the amusement of the audience, 'and almost as much as many tabloid newspaper journalists earn for writing misleading medical articles.'

'Oh, come on,' countered Carole, 'maybe a few, but not many. Most journalists earn nowhere near that amount. What annoys me most is that I had to fight tooth and nail to get my elderly mother admitted to hospital, fed properly and treated like a human being. Many doctors seem more interested in the money these days, and don't seem to care.'

Then, rather charmingly, she gently touched my arm and added, 'Present company excepted, I know *you* do. But I do feel that good doctors should earn their wages and that the best ones should be rewarded most.'

She'd just been so nice to me, it had all but taken the wind from my sails. Alan Titchmarsh continued to probe and provoke in his subtle and sensitive manner, but in reality all the heat and sting in the controversy had gone. To have a really good ding-dong in a TV debate, it is definitely better to invite two panellists who genuinely loathe each other, then you can get the live audience and viewers at home foaming at the mouth. But on this particular occasion, Carole and I didn't fit the bill. We just could not help liking each other.

11

Anabolics

BRITAIN'S OLYMPIC MEDAL HAUL IN BEIJING WAS TRULY inspirational and gripped the nation. It was such a refreshing change to hear stories of sacrifice, dedication and endeavour when television usually glories in mediocrity and humiliation. Is it really not possible to have more programmes on television that might motivate youngsters in Britain to achieve something truly brilliant for themselves? Stories like that of the mountaineer Joe Simpson, who, having nearly died after a freak climbing accident in the Peruvian Andes when he broke his leg and crawled to safety in terrible conditions, not only went on to make the film *Touching the Void* about his experience but defied doctors' advice and went on to climb other mountains and accept other challenges. Stories like that of Steve Redgrave, who won his fifth Olympic gold medal in rowing after being diagnosed and treated for Type 1 diabetes. Stories like that of Lance Armstrong, who became a professional athlete at the age of sixteen but developed testicular cancer which spread to his brain and lungs in 1996. At that time, doctors gave him a 50 per cent chance of survival. He underwent surgery twice and then had chemotherapy. Five months later, he was back on his bike and subsequently won the Tour de France on seven separate occasions. Then there is Bob Champion, the amazing jockey who also developed a male cancer in two parts of his body in 1979 and was given only a few months to live. He said that only his dream enabled him to get through the hardship of chemotherapy. In 1981, he realized that dream when he won the Grand National on Aldaniti – not only a very public victory but also a very personal one against cancer.

What about Paula Radcliffe, MBE, who has won ten world records, been the BBC's Sports Personality of the Year, and had a baby, Isla, in January 2007 before winning the New York Marathon in November of the same year in the fantastic time of two hours, twenty-two minutes and nine seconds? It is amazing to think that marathon runners of this calibre are running every hundred yards in about fifteen seconds. I personally met and was inspired by Dame Kelly Holmes, who in 2004 won an Olympic Gold in the 800 and 1,500 metres in the summer Olympics. She had already been a British Army teenage champion and won her gold medals despite a bout of depression after recurrent leg injuries which had driven her to self-harming and suicidal thoughts.

Paralympian Tanni Grey-Thompson has won fourteen medals, nine of which are gold, countless European titles, six London Marathons and holds thirty world records. She is a fantastically positive and breathtakingly honest person who once said, 'For me, it's not about pretending I don't have a disability. I'm just a very competitive person. I love finishing a hard session not being sure if I'm going to be sick or not.' And finally, I am inspired by Marlon Shirley, a paralympian who's become the fastest man on one foot and the only leg amputee to break the 11-second barrier for the 100 metres. He had been abandoned by his parents as a three-year-old and lost his foot in a lawn mower accident two years later. Despite this terrible early start in life, he was determined not to give up. To see him run on his S-shaped carbon fibre springs simply takes the breath away. If these people can achieve what they already have, who knows what other 'ordinary' people could do. They will never know until they try. We need more of this type of thing on television. But are the producers listening?

Personally, I have always enjoyed exercise and feel energized and uplifted by it. If several days go by without any fairly vigorous activity I feel slothful, lazy and mentally fat. So I suppose it isn't really surprising that over the years I have risen to the occasional sporting challenge.

'How do you fancy doing the Great North Swim and swimming a mile across Lake Windermere, Hils?' I was asked not so long ago. Anne-Marie is one of my favourite senior producers in the office, and she is constantly coming up with all sorts of brilliant ideas for the programme such as the Bikini Diet, and a campaign to get the entire nation fit before the 2012 Olympics. The Bikini Diet was a fantastic success, attracting two million hits on GMTV's website within the first two weeks and stunning everybody with its instant popularity. The idea to swim across Windermere had already been endorsed by Brendan Foster, fresh from his return from Beijing, and the plan was that Jamie Rickers, who presents our Toonattik programmes on Saturday mornings, and I would go up to Cumbria and get the ball rolling by participating in the swim with 2,000 other competitors.

Always a sucker for a sporting challenge and a bit of fun,

I rather too hastily said yes. It wouldn't be such a bad idea, I argued with myself, to get a couple of longish swims under my Speedos in the next couple of weeks, and swimming the lake with all that beautiful scenery surrounding me sounded like an opportunity not to be missed. After ploughing up and down the lovely warm pool in the spa at the Four Seasons Hotel in Dogmersfield on three or four occasions, I duly checked in at the Ambleside Hotel three weeks later. Unfortunately, it was 3.15 in the morning, and the swim was due to start in a few hours. The previous evening I'd been in Birmingham to present the New You Awards for the most outstanding progress made by members and staff of Fitness First, and I left the venue just after midnight to make the journey north. But the adrenalin was flowing and I was up for it.

Two days before this, GMTV had gone up to Windermere to where the swim was due to start, and I had talked to Mark Foster, our Olympic Gold swimmer, and to David Davies, who had come so close to winning a gold himself in Beijing in the 10K open swim. Claire Nasir had presented the weather forecast from the end of the jetty with a wonderful backdrop of brooding sky and mountains behind her.

On the morning of the swim I donned the wetsuit that had been borrowed for me, rather enjoying the silky-smooth feel of the black rubber against my skin. Ricky and I were joshing around as we mingled with the other competitors and the gallows humour at least distracted us from the prospect of immersing ourselves in that dark murky water at 15 degrees C. When the time came for our group of swimmers to start, I remember striding purposefully into the water, thinking that actually, with the wetsuit on, it didn't feel as cold as I had thought it might. But then I started to swim. As soon as I put my head in the water to swim the crawl, I had to suppress the strongest desire to inhale. The reflex to expand your lungs when hit by very cold water is immensely strong, and I remembered seeing documentaries about air-sea rescue pilots being trained to cope with emergencies in such conditions. When people are plunged into icy cold water, it is this reflex to take a deep breath which causes the death by drowning of many excellent swimmers. Unless the pilots are wearing a watertight mask that supplies air or oxygen, they stand little chance unless they can free themselves from the cockpit and get to the surface within seconds. This was exactly how I felt when I was trying to swim.

I thought I would soon become accustomed to the temperature of the water, but it kept happening. In the warm pool of the Four Seasons spa I had quickly adapted to taking three strokes with my head in the water and looking up to the left to breathe, then taking another three strokes and looking up again to breathe to the right. But here in Windermere I just could not do it. To my disgust, the only way I could breathe at all was to swim breaststroke to begin with, even though the leaders of the pack were getting further and further away. I felt a complete failure, not least because I knew the cameras behind me were rolling and the editors who would put the programme out on Monday were unlikely to spare my embarrassment. It must have taken about 400 metres, a quarter of the swim, before I could do the crawl even half efficiently, but at least the wetsuit was making me more buoyant, and I hadn't forgotten my leg kick to keep me on the move.

In a funny kind of way I enjoyed the rest of the swim, looking up occasionally to see how far behind the field I was, wondering where Jamie had got to and taking the odd peek through my goggles to see if those large pike everyone had been talking about were anywhere near. As I approached the finish, I saw various cameramen pointing their lenses in my general direction so I redoubled my efforts and hauled myself out of the water on to the slipway. But I was all over the place. I did not feel particularly tired but I couldn't run the fifty metres to the finish line without meandering crazily from left to right. In the end I was just grateful to jog across the finish and get through an interview with Mark Foster at least semi-coherently. I'd made the swim and it was a great feeling. Mark and I talked about the fun to be had and the general health benefits of swimming and in particular the Great North Swim, which we encouraged everybody to participate in whatever their level of fitness.

Everyone should be able to swim. There were people in the water that day with all kinds of disabilities, as well as able-bodied swimmers, and it was a truly inspiring day that we hoped would motivate many people to get stuck in prior to the London Olympics. After the interview I asked Mark about my not having been able to breathe.

'It takes about six or seven swims like that to get used to it,' he said. 'Luckily, I'm a sprinter and my races are all done by a hundred metres. But you do eventually get accustomed to the icy cold of the water and your breathing gets easier. Were you a bit dizzy at the end?'

'Yes,' I said, 'and I don't really know why because I didn't feel that tired.'

'It's the cold water in your ears,' he said.

Thinking about it, that made perfect sense. When ear, nose and throat specialists are investigating people with vertigo and unexplained dizziness, they perform a calorimetric test, pouring cold water into each ear in turn and then assessing balance and eye movement. Luckily, although the cold water had disorientated me, the effect had worn off within a few minutes of coming ashore.

But where was Jamie? He hadn't come in from the water yet, and Mark had told me that my time was thirty-eight minutes. When he wasn't back after an hour, we began to worry. His wife and kids didn't seem too bothered, but we were. After all, if he was going to drown or die of hypothermia, we would be expected to get it on film. I nipped behind the VIP catering tent, squeezed out of my wetsuit, pulled on some dry clothes and grabbed a beer. As I looked out of the door of the marquee, there was Jamie loping across the finishing line, a broad grin on his face. One hour, twenty-four minutes. Rubbish. But at least he was alive.

Swimming in Lake Windermere had been a new experience for me as my usual exercise consisted of running, squash, gym work and kicking a rugger ball around with the kids. I had successfully completed the New York Marathon and several local half-marathons for charity in the past, but a few years ago I had the dubious distinction of being officially banned from the London Marathon. I had previously run it in just under four hours and on this occasion I was intending to do it in half an hour less. I had been offered a VIP place and did not even have to apply for a much-sought-after entry. My twenty-seven-year-old son Seb, on the other hand, had had to apply through the usual channels, although he was a lot younger and fitter than me. Two weeks before the race, however, I developed 'shin splints', a condition which I knew would not be better in time for me to compete. Seb had not been among the one in three runners to obtain entry, so I immediately thought that he could run in my place. Why not? He was a much better runner anyway and capable of running a sub-three-hour marathon (as he subsequently proved in Amsterdam when he ran the amazing time of two hours and fifty-eight minutes). I phoned the race organizers to suggest this but they said it was not possible to transfer a race number to someone else. Why? I asked. Because you can't, they said. Computer says no.

I thought about this long and hard. Seb was keen and talented and really wanted to run. I had run the race before and could not run. All the sponsors I had arranged, who had promised money for charity, were more than happy to sponsor Seb instead. Who would know? What harm could come of it? The little bit of a rebel and the sports enthusiast in me told me just to go ahead quietly and let Seb run in my place. I would bet we were by no means the first to do it. I didn't want to upset the race organizers and I realize what we did was strictly against the rules, but it was either me failing to turn up and letting all my sponsors down, or giving Seb the opportunity to enjoy running the marathon and raise money for important causes himself. We tried to find some other way of allowing Seb to run legitimately, but without success, so we made the decision that he would simply run with my number.

Unfortunately, Seb ran extremely well and came second in the VIP category – a situation neither of us had foreseen – and the cat was out of the bag. Everybody could see that this young, talented, handsome athlete was not Dr Hilary. But the response of the race organizers was surprising in its severity. At a press conference following the marathon, a very large, overweight lawyer announced that Seb and I would be banned from future marathons and that we had compromised the safety of participants by creating a situation whereby anybody who might suffer a medical problem would not be immediately identifiable. What rubbish. Sebastian is half my age and much less likely to suffer a medical problem anyway. And what about all those hundreds of runners dressed in gorilla outfits and duck suits who risk dehydration and hyperthermia by competing over twenty-six miles when they cannot lose body heat? In my view this was not a problem associated with medical issues, it was a gut reaction to somebody riding roughshod over their regulations.

The press gleefully reported the incident and my friends and media colleagues were hugely amused. On *Have I Got News for You* the following week, Ian Hislop said, 'He can now run the London Marathon on three hundred and sixty-four days of the year, and come first every time.' As it happens, I am quite happy to have been banned from a twenty-six-mile race that I probably would never have run in again anyway. Running both the London and New York marathons had been fantastic experiences but there were plenty of new sporting challenges to which I wanted to turn my attention and energy.

As a doctor, I have always been a fervent advocate of the medical benefits of exercise. People who exercise regularly are generally more in tune with their bodies and how they feel and function. They are likely to be more aware of muscle tension, stiffness and reduced fluidity of movement when exercise has not been taken for a while. People who are fitter from regular physical activity report the ability to think faster and more clearly. They feel better in themselves and have sharper, more acute reflexes. Research has proved that regular exercise lowers the risk of heart attacks and strokes. It lowers the blood pressure and cholesterol levels. It reduces the risk of blood clots. It keeps your weight down naturally. It prevents brittle bone disease and reduces the risk of diabetes. It improves the quality of sleep and mood, reducing anxiety and depression and neutralizing stress.

171

It has also been shown to lessen the risk of certain cancers.

Many people who take up a sport feel so good that they go on to exercise excessively. They spend inordinate amounts of time in the gym, at the expense of their work and social life. This is because the neurotransmitters, endorphins, which are produced as a result of exercise are like opiates in the brain. They give the person a buzz and a wonderful sense of euphoria. As in all things, moderation is the key. But I personally have no doubt that if more people exercised regularly, we would see far less illness in the surgery, fewer prescriptions for pharmaceutical medication and much slimmer and happier people in general. In the future, I would love to pioneer a national network of exercise clinics and mobile gyms run by doctors to get the nation healthier and fitter. But knowing how the authorities in the UK and their sedentary lawyers work, I am sure it would be banned before it even got off the ground.

I feel passionate about the health benefits of exercise and take every opportunity to pass this advice on to anyone who will listen. But there's one question I often get back in return: to what extent does regular physical activity really prolong your life? Recently I got the chance to ask a man who might know. At a conference on cardiology which I had had to attend in order to pass my compulsory annual GP appraisal, I was talking to an eminent London professor about the benefits of exercise for a healthy heart. To be honest, the professor looked way older than his years and as if he'd never taken a day's exercise in his life.

'There's no doubt,' he said rather pompously. 'Regular aerobic exercise of thirty minutes' duration taken three times a week is likely to extend your life by an average of two years.'

'Is that all?' I asked.

'Yes,' he said. 'But if you add up all those thirty-minute sessions throughout your life, you'll find that it comes to about two years anyway. So unless you actually enjoy going to the gym or pounding the streets, I really can't see any point to it.'

It was an interesting opinion and one which made me laugh out loud. But I couldn't help feeling that this was wishful thinking on his part rather than being based on any scientific evidence. My view was sadly confirmed when the poor old boy subsequently dropped dead of a heart attack at the tender age of fifty-four.

The trick, I think, is to ensure that the exercise you take is enjoyable, varied and fun. And that the potential health benefits are not ruined by relying on anything artificial or unnatural such as creatine-enriched high protein meal replacements or hormone supplements in the form of anabolic steroids. In fact, I once recorded an interesting little TV programme designed to make this very point. I had been working with Trevor, my cameraman, Ali Lutz, one of our best producers, and Jack, the sound man, on a series of 'one-minute TV', a commercially sponsored set of mini films based, in this case, on summer health. We'd been down to Lasham Flying School to do a piece on fear of flying, we'd been to Whitewater Nursery, the local garden centre, to talk about plant allergies and we'd discussed hay fever, sunburn and a good first-aid kit for travellers on the beach in Bournemouth. We'd worked hard and had plenty of footage in the can, but decided to do one more piece for fun although we imagined it would never be broadcast.

'I know,' I said. 'I wrote this poem a little while ago about the side effects of anabolic steroids. You know, the ones that athletes take. The ones that more and more young kids are taking as they become more freely available in gyms up and down the country. Most people have no idea about what they do. Let's do it as a rap song, with me in costume looking the part, and I can't sing anyway.'

'Perfect,' said Trev. 'Anything for a laugh.'

Ali, however, was not so sure.

'It's a bit off the subject, isn't it?' she said.

'I don't know,' I replied. 'In the summer loads more people want to shape up and get fit and lots of them go down to the gym and try to take short cuts to get a fantastic physique artificially. Anabolic steroids are rife right now, and people just don't realize how dangerous they can be. People are taking one steroid to bulk up their muscles, another to harden them, and a third to burn fat so they look more defined. They call it "stacking" but it's illegal and hazardous. Anabolic steroids make your hair fall out, enlarge your heart, damage your kidneys, cause masculinization in women and prostate cancer, testicular shrinkage and infertility in men. Young people don't know all this, but if we do it as a rap song they might just sit up and take notice.'

Ali raised her eyes to the heavens, but since we'd got plenty of material already she agreed to go along with it. We pinched a suitable non-copyright backing track from the music library and negotiated a couple of hours of time to film at Beechdown, my local squash club and gym. We took our camera down there the following day. We had oiled up Simon, one of the personal trainers there, who looked muscular and 'ripped', and I donned some rapper gear, switched on the CD backing track and began jumping about. We did it in one take, with me preceding the song by saying that the use of anabolic steroids could seriously damage your health. 'Let me put that in a language that young people can easily understand,' I said, and with Simon pumping iron in the background, I started:

He's a body builder, he got legs like iron. Got the broadest
   shoulders that the broads just love to cry on.
His pecs are quite fantastic, so hard defined and cut. He got a
   washboard stomach and a corrugated gut.
He used to train Ben Johnson but Ben Johnson went and blew it.
   He takes a lot of steroids but he really shouldn't do it.
Anabolics, bolics, bolics. Anabolics, bolics, bolics.
He loves to flex his biceps, his lats and triceps too, he loves to
   pose without no clothes and pull a bird or two.
He takes them back to his place where he works out for an hour
   and then they plead for sex with him with strength and
   staying power.
But when they pull his kit off, they can't believe their eyes.
   There's stretch marks on his buttocks and huge veins across
   his thighs.
Anabolics, bolics, bolics. Anabolics, bolics, bolics.
All this damn testosterone has made him such a hunk, but then
   they see regrettably his private parts have shrunk.
They soon no longer see him as a general factotum, just a
   balding body builder with a sad and shrivelled scrotum.
They knock him round the room a bit, they hurt him with cruel
   jokes, and that is why he's cowering in this place for battered
   blokes.
Admission here's restricted just for body-building nomads with
   hard-to-find appendages and microscopic gonads.
Anabolics, bolics, bolics. Anabolics, bolics, bolics.

At the end, I looked down the lens of the camera and said,
'Well, I hope that's clear enough: just say no to anabolic
steroids. Simon here has built his fantastic physique the hard
way, naturally and cleanly without drugs, so if you want to
stay fit and healthy, make sure you do the same.'
   We edited the piece back at the studio, where Dean, one

of our most creative editors, applied some fantastic black and white flashy bits with a highly technical piece of kit called a Quantel Paintbox. We never imagined in a million years that it would be aired, and just forgot about it.

Of the twenty little pieces on summer health which we completed, only six were ever broadcast. Anabolics was one of them and, to our utter amazement, not a single complaint has yet been received about either the content or my terrible singing. Maybe the lawyers are still working on what charges to bring.

12

Thin Women, Thin Lips, Thin Evidence

IT WAS ALL OVER THE NEWS THAT FERN BRITTON HAD HAD gastric surgery and had lost weight artificially rather than by means of the healthy food and exercise she had previously claimed were responsible. Most of the newspapers and apparently many of their readers were calling her a cheat.

I felt sorry for Fern. She is one of the most professional, entertaining, humorous and genuinely warm presenters I have ever met, and who knows what private misery drove her to take the huge step of undergoing the surgeon's knife when clearly nothing else she had tried had worked. Following her gastric banding, she had lost five stone and had dropped several dress sizes, and was seen wearing sleeveless dresses with a belt around her waist. She looked all the happier for it. But inevitably newspaper commentators and others, perhaps jealous of her new-found figure, were quick to criticize the action she had taken.

Bariatric surgery, which includes stomach stapling, gastric banding and bypass operations, undoubtedly works when used appropriately. Gastric banding, occasionally referred to as 'lap banding', is a very effective procedure to help over-weight people achieve considerable long-term weight loss. It works by restricting the amount of food a person can eat and is most successful for individuals who eat large-volume meals. Research shows that, on average, people who undergo gastric banding will lose around half of their excess weight within two years of surgery. The average actual weight loss is about half a stone a month, although this obviously varies between patients.

A gastric bypass, on the other hand, works by reducing the size of the stomach by bypassing it altogether. This operation is most successful for patients who snack and eat a lot of chocolate. The average weight loss for this procedure is 70 per cent of the excess weight within a year. Other celebrities known to have benefited from such procedures include X Factor's Sharon Osbourne, footballer Diego Maradona, TV comedienne Roseanne Barr and TV presenter Anne Diamond. Anne had been heavily criticized for being less than generous with the truth about her surgery prior to competing in Celebrity Fit Club.

The whole debate raised a number of interesting issues. What were the genuine medical benefits of such procedures? What were the cosmetic advantages? What were the side effects and risks? And did all this publicity about celebrity patients open the floodgates for millions of other people demanding inappropriate gastric banding on the NHS?

The medical benefits are clear. The health risks associated with obesity itself are widely recognized. It significantly increases the risk of heart attacks and strokes. The risk of Type 2 diabetes is eighty times higher in people whose body mass index exceeds 40. Other studies have shown the relationship between obesity and premature death and even some cancers, such as gullet, thyroid, kidney, colon and endometrial cancers.

Even moderate weight loss leads to major improvements in blood pressure, cholesterol levels and blood sugar levels. Relief from back and joint pain, breathlessness and sleep apnoea is also dramatic. But other methods of weight loss can achieve the same results, albeit less dramatically. So what criteria need to be satisfied before anyone should be considered for bariatric surgery?

Responsible guidelines dictate that it can be considered in people with a BMI over 40, or over 35 if a patient also has an obesity-related disease. The patient should have tried other weight loss treatments first, there should be no psychological reason for the obesity and the patient should fully understand the lifestyle changes that such surgery will entail. When seeking help in the first place, anyone contemplating surgery should be fully assessed by a specialist dietician or bariatric nurse before talking to the surgeon. Patients should then be followed up by their consultants three, six and twelve months after their operation and have one-to-one follow-ups with a dietician every month for at least a year.

Carole Malone, my *News of the World* fellow columnist, lost her excess weight the hard way and did extremely well. Whenever I see her in the TV studio, I make a point of complimenting her on how brilliantly she has done in maintaining her new shape. But I know she is really concerned about how many miserable, grossly overweight women are now looking at Fern or Anne and thinking the only effective way to slim down is to go under the surgeon's knife.

In the GMTV studio, mother of two Kerry De Ste Croix came in to tell us about the downside of her gastric bypass. She had hers done when she weighed twenty-one stone and paid £9,000 to have the operation privately. But while she is now a svelte ten stone, she was very keen to tell people about the negative psychological impact of her surgery. Since her operation, she had found eating almost any food impossible as it made her sick. Her stomach was now the size of an egg. The range of food she could eat was very restricted and some people, she said, felt faint and sweaty after eating sugary foods as a result of something called 'dumping' syndrome, where rapid stomach emptying leads to fluid being drawn into the intestine from the blood, resulting in changes in blood pressure and blood sugar levels.

Other medical dangers include damage to other organs during surgery, for which the mortality rate is a not in-considerable 1 in 2,000. The access port used to inject saline into the gastric band to adjust it can develop a leak and necessitate minor surgery to correct it. If the band is not properly fitted, patients can suffer from reflux of stomach acid causing heartburn and aspiration pneumonia. The opening between the two stomach pouches can become blocked by food, requiring an operation to unblock it. For the first four weeks after the procedure, a strict liquid-only diet is vital and gallstones are more likely in anyone losing weight quickly because the gall bladder contracts less frequently than it used to.

Bariatric surgery has a place, but it can never be com-pletely safe and it is not always free of long-term side effects. Before people reach the stage where their body mass index rises beyond 30, steps should be taken to rein in calorie intake and increase exercise levels. There is still no quick-fix route to weight loss, and despite all the hype about break-through treatments the healthier lifestyle option is still the best and safest. Nor do weight loss medications, very low calorie diets or surgery confront the underlying psychological reasons for the overeating, which remain present after the treatment is discontinued.

The side effects of slimming medication can be horrendous. Who wants to take xenical, for example, and suffer from faecal incontinence? Who fancies taking sibutramine and not sleeping at night while shaking and feeling anxious all day? The licence for Rimonabant has already been temporarily suspended for overweight people with metabolic syndrome because of links with depression. So why don't more people realize that the time to do something about their weight gain is before it gets out of hand in the first place? I know it is a complex issue and that reaching this ideal is easier said than done. But with the right help from dedicated health professionals, personal trainers, nutritionists and life coaches, coupled with better public facilities for fun exercise, there is no reason why millions of people could not become slimmer and fitter as well as a lot healthier.

Cosmetic surgery is enjoying a boom period. Despite the recession, tens of thousands of men and women are spending the money they would ordinarily have saved for a holiday or a new car on breast implants, nose jobs, facelifts and liposuction. Botox injections are performed for groups of people at social functions, lip plumping is de rigueur and collagen fillers and laser resurfacing are all the rage.

But is cosmetic surgery all it is cracked up to be? For many, a straightforward operation can change their lives completely. A woman who has no libido because of a completely flat chest can rediscover her sexuality and, for the first time in her life, happily initiate lovemaking with her partner because of her new-found confidence. Someone very self-conscious about the size of their nose or the saggy skin around their middle after drastic weight loss or childbirth can derive a terrific psychological boost from an aesthetic procedure to correct it.

On the other hand, having cosmetic breast surgery simply because your boyfriend wants you to look like Jordan or because you are slightly dissatisfied with some minor imperfection or, even worse, *lots* of minor imperfections, is likely to lead to disappointment. There have been many well-documented cases of tragedies occurring where cosmetic surgery has gone wrong. Many a patient has returned from surgery overseas, having believed it to be a cheaper option, only to report highly unsatisfactory results with no legal comeback.

Denise Hendry, wife of Scottish football international Colin Hendry, had her bowel perforated several times during a liposuction procedure, and I interviewed a thirty-year-old man on breakfast TV about his horrific experiences in a cosmetic surgery clinic in South Africa. Persuaded by a friend while he was on holiday to lose his paunch, he was literally cut open from one side of his waist to the other, leaving an ugly puckered scar two feet long. The cosmetic result was appalling, he had been left in a lot of pain and to add insult to injury he had heard nursing staff laughing about his stupidity in having the operation in the first place while he recovered from his anaesthetic in the corridor. He had no means under international law of making a formal complaint and no British surgeon – either NHS or private – had any interest in correcting some other butcher's work. It was a sobering piece and hopefully one which would make many people contemplating such drastic action on a whim think twice.

I always tell anybody considering such surgery to think

very carefully beforehand. Will the operation really improve how they feel about themselves? Or will they become a serial patient, always craving another nip here or a tuck there yet never being truly happy? Would a counsellor or psychotherapist be a more appropriate source of help?

However, provided a patient has thought carefully about all the options and the operation is reasonable, I am happy to refer them to a surgeon I know who has the experience and expertise required. I believe all patients should be counselled at length by the surgeon intending to perform the operation too. Patients need to know that results can never be guaranteed and that side effects of the operation can occur, such as bruising, swelling, scarring and infection. It is vital that the surgeon is registered with a professional specialist body such as the BAAPS (British Association of Aesthetic Plastic Surgeons) or BACS (British Association of Cosmetic Surgeons) and has professional indemnity in case something goes wrong.

Finding a surgeon through an advertisement in Yellow Pages or elsewhere is always dodgy, although going by word of mouth to a surgeon recommended by somebody who is highly satisfied with their results and aftercare is reasonable. Good surgeons with plenty of experience are usually very happy to put potential clients in touch with previous patients and to show before-and-after photographs of their surgery. Some even use computer-generated images to give the client a better idea of how they may look after the operation.

I always warn people about the risks of going abroad for surgery just because it is cheaper. I have seen many patients return from Poland and other parts of the EU, having had surgery performed by inexperienced, jobbing locum surgeons who have disfigured them for life. I am also suspicious of surgeons offering discounts if, say, a boob job is combined with liposuction, where the patient had never previously contemplated the second operation. The cosmetic surgery industry will have to police itself more carefully if it wishes to remain as unregulated as it currently is. Having said that, the results of good cosmetic surgery in expert hands can be fantastic and it can revolutionize people's lives.

For me, however, vaginal rejuvenation seems a step too far. In a recent edition of the *British Journal of Sexual Medicine*, a review of designer vaginoplasty amused me greatly. Apparently, the lips around your mouth are not the only ones you can have treated. There has been a rise in the popularity of American gynaecologists who can shorten the length of your labia or the laxity of your love lips. A certain Dr David Matlock, known also as Dr Sex, reckons to have pioneered laser vaginal rejuvenation and regularly carries out liposculpture 'down below'. It seems he is now a multi-millionaire, with clients paying up to £41,000 to have their bits made neater or more symmetrical. One of his rivals even dubbed himself 'the Genitailor' just in case anyone was in doubt as to how he earned his living.

Jessica Brinton, writing in *The Times* online, says of Matlock, 'He sees his role as one of liberating women from the tyranny of sexual inadequacy and disappointment. By arming us with the tools for total physical dominion over our private parts he is to his mind setting us free.' Ha. Other surgeons perform such procedures as the 'G-Shot', a collagen injection placed below the Grafenberg Spot to make it easier to find and hopefully more sensitive.

Laser vaginal rejuvenation is intended to tighten muscles stretched by childbirth and to prevent or treat urinary incontinence and loss of sensation. But the medical jury is still out on whether this type of cosmetic surgery is justified

184

at all. One Beverly Hills plastic surgeon has allegedly criticized Dr Matlock by saying that he has never in his life heard a man say, 'I saw this woman, she had an ugly vagina,' and that Matlock is therefore promoting dysmorphophobia – a psychological condition where a patient is obsessed with the imperfections of their own body. It has been suggested that in France this type of surgery could attract a popular following and catch on nationally. The French government, it seems, is already very happy to pay for every woman who wants it to have ten sessions of physiotherapy for pelvic floor tightening after giving birth. Great. Good old President Sarkozy. Watch out, Carla Bruni.

Maybe if we all took a little more care of ourselves, there would be less need for cosmetic surgery. If our lifestyles were healthier, maybe we would see less of doctors altogether. And if we availed ourselves of DIY diagnostic testing possibly we could dispense with them completely. This was the subject of a recent *Tonight* programme with Trevor McDonald. They had lined up five old school chums and subjected them to a battery of self-testing kits freely available over the counter at high street chemists, including cholesterol, blood glucose and liver function tests. The commercial market for these products is now worth £99 million per annum, and it is a growing and lucrative business attracting a great deal of interest. But is it worth the money, is it reliable and can it either worry people unnecessarily if the results are unfavourable or, worse still, make them complacent if the result is falsely negative? Can it even be dangerous if it fails to pick up something serious, or drives people to do something silly if they find a result which is shocking?

There are all kinds of DIY tests these days. Tests on the urine for sugar, protein, chlamydia and pregnancy. Tests on the blood for diabetes, liver disease and heart disease. You can measure your own nicotine and alcohol levels, blood pressure and body fat composition. You can analyse your drinks to see if they have been spiked at a nightclub, send off fingerprick blood samples for food intolerances, blow into peak flow meters to assess asthma severity, and carry out assessments of your own future fertility.

The *Tonight* programme invited me to come up to a school in Luton to meet the five ex-classmates and to interpret and comment on the results of their tests. The samples had also been simultaneously analysed by an accredited BUPA laboratory using sophisticated and quality-controlled technology, and these results were available to us as well. As we gathered in the main school hall for the filming, the little group of five looked nervous and apprehensive as they waited to hear news of their health checks.

Many of the results were accurate when compared to the BUPA tests, and most were reassuringly normal. But a surprisingly high proportion were significantly outside the normal acceptable range for adults of their age, and several recorded dramatically different readings when compared to the more reliable laboratory analysis. Three of the group, who had used at least two different kinds of over-the-counter test kits, had blood sugar levels suggesting they had diabetes. Laboratory testing showed they did not. One had recorded such a low level of blood sugar that, had it been true, he would have been unconscious in a hypoglycaemic coma. On cholesterol testing, three of them posted desirable levels of blood fats, whereas the BUPA tests showed that in fact they were on the highish side.

The televised chat we had was interesting because it revealed how difficult our guinea pigs had found it to follow the instructions in the test kits, and how puzzled they remained when the results were compared to the hospital tests. We talked about why the results were sometimes so different, and how it could possibly happen. We discussed the vagaries of the finger-pricking technique, which most of them had found surprisingly difficult to perform on themselves, and how a drop of blood squeezed vigorously out of a fingertip and left so long that it begins to clot before it is analysed might give a false reading. We debated how hit and miss it could be to read off a result by referring to a graded colour chart similar to a Dulux paint chart. All in all, the consensus of opinion among the five ex-classmates was that they probably wouldn't bother using these DIY tests if they had to buy them themselves. They would certainly want to visit their doctor to discuss the results afterwards, which would rather defeat the object of the exercise.

But *Tonight* did give me the chance to say that DIY tests still have a place, and Dr Chris Steele of *This Morning* fame agreed with me. He went as far as to say that DIY testing had actually saved lives and would do so in the future. I mentioned that of the 2.3 million diabetics in the UK, up to 500,000 were still not diagnosed. Since health care professionals were still not picking them up through screening, DIY testing at least offered them the opportunity to detect the disease for themselves. In doing so, it would prevent progressive damage to their eyes, heart and kidneys which in time costs the NHS so many billions trying to treat, and ultimately claims so many lives. Surely it is better, we argued, to at least have an idea of your cholesterol number, or how much your liver is struggling to cope with the amount of fat you eat or alcohol you drink?

Yet interpretation of the results is everything. The manufacturers' leaflets and explanations which accompany the testing kits are short and simplified. The disclaimer at the bottom and the recommendation to visit your doctor is half-hearted and confined to the small print. For an industry worth £99 million a year, the *Tonight* programme concluded that it would have to improve the accuracy of its testing and provide customers with a much more readily available source of advice when needed.

A few weeks before the *Tonight* programme, I'd been doing an interview with a very young and rather inexperienced-sounding presenter from a radio station down in Pembrokeshire on this very same subject of do-it-yourself diagnostic testing. I was at Radio Lynx in Fulham talking down an ISDN line. I was telling the presenter about a new DIY urine-testing kit that people could obtain over the counter at the chemist and check themselves out with. But he simply didn't get it. He couldn't seem to grasp the importance of such a test and kept on asking me the same question over and over again about what it could do. An explanation about the possible abnormal presence of red cells, white cells, bacteria or protein in the urine sample made him none the wiser. It was like banging my head against a brick wall. Then I was struck by a thought: he's young, he's a bloke, he's Welsh, and the All Black rugby team are currently touring the UK. You have to know your audience in this game, and I hoped this spark of an idea I'd had was going to work.

'Do you play rugby?' I asked.

'Is the Pope Catholic?' came the reply.

'Well, you know the All Blacks are touring the UK right now?'

'Oh yes.'

'And you know Jonah Lomu?'

'Oh yes. Their best player.'

'And that he's had a kidney transplant that has kept him out of the team?'

'I read something about that.'

'Well, that condition is called nephrotic syndrome, where large amounts of protein are lost in the urine because of inflammation and disease in the kidney.'

'Crikey.'

'So if he'd used a DIY testing kit like this when he first started to feel ill or, more importantly, several months before he started to feel ill, his illness might never have become so serious, and he might even have been playing against Cardiff on Saturday.'

Pause.

'That's amazing, that is. So this testing kit is fantastic then? I hope all the Welsh boys are using it. What's it called again? We'll do a special promo for our listeners . . .'

Looking through the glass window of the sound booth from where I was broadcasting, I could see the girl from the PR agency positively beaming with pleasure. This was one radio interview the client would definitely be receiving in DVD form later.

13

Fear of Flying

THERE IS NOTHING LIKE A STIFF GIN AND TONIC TO OVER-come a fear of flying. On top of a 40mg tablet of propranolol your nerves are calm, your hands no longer shake, your palms are dry once more, your stomach settled and all those nasty palpitations are replaced by a wonderful feeling of peace and serenity as you gaze out of the aeroplane window at all those white fluffy clouds just below you. Propranolol is a beta-blocker, a type of medication also used for the reduction of high blood pressure, angina, migraine and abnormal heart rhythms, which works by blocking the action of powerful stress hormones like noradrenalin. Unlike more powerful anxiolytics such as Valium and Librium, it neutralizes all the physical effects of anxiety without causing much sedation and so allows people's brains to function quite normally. This is why it is such a good medication for people terrified at the prospect of after-dinner speaking or flying. The gin element of my own treatment for fear of flying is just the icing on the cake. If you have overcome the mental apprehension, why not go

190

one step further and enjoy the whole experience in a state of happy euphoria? I know I do.

Yet apparently one in six airline passengers endures the hell of aerophobia while never admitting to it as they do not want to appear weak and pathetic. For those most severely affected, however, the terror can be so bad it paralyses them and renders them incapable of boarding the plane. This holds true even if it means missing their child's wedding or the family holiday of a lifetime. The statistics tell us that flying is hundreds of times safer than driving anywhere in a car or even walking down the street but, as with other phobias, the fear is totally irrational. You cannot reason it away. Various airlines, however, run very effective courses designed to overcome fear of flying and the vast majority of people who go on them successfully master their phobia and cope perfectly well with flying thereafter. The course usually involves some CBT – cognitive behavioural therapy – in which experienced pilots explain how aeroplanes stay up in the sky and what all the different engine noises actually signify. The session generally finishes with a pleasant and relaxed flight around the airport and nearby, and a lovely time is had by all. I'm not sure whether gin and propranolol is provided, but I somehow doubt it.

I was thinking about all this recently while flying to Lapland with the wonderful charity Northern Lights, which was taking about twenty young children with life-threatening conditions to visit Santa in the Arctic Circle. A wedding party on board the same flight included an elderly lady of about eighty. When she complained to the flight attendant that she felt a little strange, she was moved further down the plane to a seat opposite me that offered her considerably more legroom as it was adjacent to an exit. As I sat chatting to her I could see that she was about to faint.

191

Sweat formed on her upper lip and brow, her eyes glazed over, she started slurring her words and she swayed. I just managed to catch her before she pitched forward, unconscious. Gently I laid her out on the floor of the cabin and placed her feet up on a seat. It was clear she was away with the fairies and she was twitching slightly. But it was hardly surprising. It turned out that she was wearing not two but three woollen cardigans as well as a blouse and whatever she had on underneath, plus thick winter leggings. I think most people would have fainted from the heat generated by wearing all that. Asking the flight attendant for the aircraft's medical bag and praying we were not going to have to divert the plane for an emergency landing, I checked her pulse, blood pressure, respiration rate and pupils. All good, but her skin was very cool and clammy and she still looked ghostly white. By the time we had removed the cardigans, however, she was starting to come round. I used the equipment in the medical bag to check her over and rule out a stroke or a heart attack. Within minutes she was back in her seat and fully restored, if rather embarrassed and self-conscious about what had happened. She needn't be, I reassured her.

As the flight attendant was still loitering nearby, I summoned, in the most authoritative voice I could muster, a large gin and tonic with ice and lemon.

'For the passenger who fainted?' she asked.

'Absolutely not. For me,' I said. 'I'm the one who needs it most.'

And off she scuttled to the galley to fetch it. Result. It wasn't quite the heroic and potentially life-saving procedure that had been carried out by Professor Angus Wallace some months before, though. He'd been a passenger aboard a flight from Hong Kong to London and had used a metal coat hanger and brandy bottle to revive another in-flight patient who had suffered a tension pneumothorax. In this condition, a burst lung allows inhaled air to escape into the chest cavity, which slowly builds up pressure, collapses the lung and pushes the heart and mediastinum over to the other side. This becomes a serious medical emergency capable of causing death by asphyxiation and cardiac arrest. It's not on record whether the good prof was ever rewarded with a giant gin and tonic, but if the airline had had any decency, a chilled jeroboam of Krug would surely not, in my humble opinion, have been inappropriate.

On the hairiest flight I have ever been on – and I've been on a few – gin and tonic was not even on board. Many years ago, when I was working for a company called Offshore Medical Support in the Shetlands, I was part of the on-duty medical team attending a girl who had been brought in having uncontrollable seizures. The girl's body convulsed as wave after wave of muscular contractions swept over her fragile frame. Her teeth bit down on her tongue to cause bloodstained frothing at the mouth, her bladder voided itself involuntarily as her abdominal muscles forcibly contracted and her limbs thrashed around wildly in the unmistakable tonic-clonic dance of grand mal epilepsy. Only this was not a normal seizure. Normal seizures usually settle quickly, within two or three minutes, and leave the patient sleepy and confused. This was different. This girl's convulsions kept hitting her repeatedly, every two or three minutes, giving her no time to recover and threatening her brain with oxygen starvation. This was status epilepticus, a life-threatening condition I'd only ever seen once before in a fully staffed casualty department.

The girl looked about twenty or twenty-one with pale

skin and shoulder-length mousy hair. She was obviously a local girl living in one of the small crofts around the Sullom Voe oil refinery and she had been brought to British Petroleum's small hospital there because an agreement existed with the local GPs that emergencies requiring evacuation for specialist treatment would be organized with our help. As one of the doctors there, I had put up an intravenous drip and given several bolus doses of diazepam already but it had made little difference. We had taken blood in order to determine at a later date the exact cause of the convulsions, but there was no Medic Alert or similar medical identity tag suggesting that she was a previous sufferer. We had no history to go on and we had no clue as to the circumstances surrounding the seizures. There was talk of magic mushroom abuse in the area, where youngsters would boil up the wild mushrooms and then drink the top of the resulting liquid to give them hallucinogenic experiences, and this was certainly one of many possibilities we were considering. But whatever the cause of the seizures, right now getting this girl flown to Aberdeen as soon as possible would be the best hope of stabilizing her and possibly saving her life.

As the doctor on duty that night, I would travel with her. I was not looking forward to it as there was a force-eight gale blowing, which often happens in Shetland. Rain was coming down horizontally and it was icy cold. The Range Rover ambulance got us to our immediate destination within twenty minutes. Scatsta was a disused RAF airfield that had served as a base in the war. The runway was short and ran north–south. Taking off in this direction in a blustery force-eight westerly was going to be far from ideal. My heart sank further when a tired rusty-looking Islander aircraft was rolled out of the airfield's only hangar. The twin-prop aircraft was designed for island-hopping and specially adapted to perform emergency landings on beaches such as Foula when the tide was out. I could immediately see several areas on the plane's fuselage where the paint had peeled off, and loose, rusting rivets somehow seemed to be holding the wings together. It was clear we would not be flying business class.

Moments later I had my patient strapped down on a stretcher at the back of the plane with her intravenous drip running and a medical bag of tricks by my side. As the pilot asked me in his strong Scottish accent if I was ready, the engines roared and we hurtled down the runway. Lurching from left to right, the Islander launched itself upwards after what seemed like a mere hundred yards, only to be thrown around crazily in the turbulence. The engine noise was tremendous and induced another convulsion in my very sick patient. Turning up the intravenous drip to provide her with yet more anti-convulsant, I suddenly became aware of a fusillade of noise from the outside of the plane. Ominously loud cracking sounds were coming from all along its fuselage. *Thump. Thwack. Crash.* The plane seemed to be tearing itself apart. I had never heard anything like this before. The plane rocked upwards before falling again and the pilot was struggling to keep it level. But the cracking noises on the outside just got worse. It felt as if the plane was falling to bits, ripped open by the elements, and at that moment I was convinced the three of us were going to die. I must have looked terrified too, as I peered out of the window at the heavy black clouds tugging at the wings and the sheets of rain rushing by in the pale moonlight. As I turned back, the pilot was looking at me steadily.

'Ach, dinnae mind yerself wi that,' he said calmly. 'Just a

wee bit ice comin aff them propellers, see. Kenwit Ah mean? Ah wudnae worry boot it.'

Amazingly, he didn't look at all concerned. Apparently this was normal. I redoubled my efforts with the girl and within moments of the Islander dragging itself free of the top level of cloud the crashing noises ceased, the turbulence abated and we were cruising much more comfortably across the North Sea towards Aberdeen. Now I experienced the adrenalin rush, that euphoric and unique feeling you get when you really appreciate life after moments of danger. Adventurers often say that you never feel completely alive until you have put yourself in danger and risked losing your life. It is certainly an interesting paradox. Up there in that vintage and noisy aeroplane with a young and very ill patient by my side and a dour Scotsman at the controls, I felt that euphoria after danger for maybe the first time. And I understood it.

I have since thought that it must be the sensation that makes doctors, nurses and paramedics working in emergency medicine so motivated to do what they do. With every helicopter rescue at sea, every road accident victim scraped off the road and ferried to the roof of a major hospital for emergency treatment and with every potholing disaster, the rescuers are aware that they are taking significant risks in order to save another human being. In a way they are flirting with fate and the only consolation they have is that their training, their skills and their discipline are more than likely to get them through it. My experience was all the more rewarding for the fact that our patient made a full recovery after specialist treatment on the Scottish mainland and was happily brought home a few days later. The exact cause of her convulsions was never discovered but she showed no lasting ill effects and that at least was a blessing.

The following day I had my reward. The pilot invited me to sit upfront with him on the way home and gave me an impromptu flying lesson, casually instructing me as I manipulated the joystick and flew between the soft white fluffy clouds down the west coast of Shetland. It was one of those rare beautiful days in that part of the world with the air swept clean by the storm and the sea a deep azure blue and shimmering like a mirror. Below us were the huge crude-oil carriers ploughing their way backwards and forwards to the Sullom Voe oil terminal to pick up cargo. Over to our right, cruising just above the waves, was the smaller spotter plane used to keep watch on the tankers to make sure they were not discharging their tanks into the sea. The deserted broad sandy beaches off Scalloway, Walls and Sanderness looked beautiful but I could see the huge breakers from the north Atlantic swell smashing against the jagged rocks. Once again that adrenalin rush. This was what working in medicine could sometimes give you. The endless conveyor belt of sore throats, boils and tummy pains in the surgery might be our bread and butter, but this was so different. It was a magically satisfying moment. It felt good to be alive.

As pleasant as this complimentary flying lesson was, however, I am reliably informed that the ultimate in-flight euphoria comes not from a miniature bottle of gin nor from piloting a light aircraft over the beautiful Shetland coastline on a clear day. I am told it comes from satisfying the entry requirements of the Mile High Club. By definition, membership is open to anyone who has enjoyed sexual congress in an aeroplane flying at a height of at least 5,280 feet above the ground. Does this mean that making love at 5,279 feet doesn't count? I don't know. But it would seem harsh.

According to a recent article in the *British Journal of Sexual Medicine*, couples intent on attaining the necessary criteria to join the club will perform under airline blankets, rendezvous in unattended galleys during long flights, and become temporary contortionists in the tight confines of the nearest lavatory. According to Wikipedia, the first ever member of the Mile High Club was Lawrence Sperry, who apparently embarked on sexual activity with a suitable female while piloting his Curtiss flying boat in November 1916. These days I assume his membership would be revoked as they were only flying at a height of 500 feet before the plane crashed – not fatally, as it happens, as they landed on water – while his mind was elsewhere. It is a matter of pure speculation whether the subsequent development of autopilot technology at the Sperry Corporation, a famous electrical equipment and electronics company, was related to this incident or just a coincidence.

For many, the rare opportunity to lie back, sample an in-flight meal and enjoy a good book or a film is quite sufficient. And as the travel writer Rolf Potts says on the internet, 'Aspiring to have sex on a commercial flight is now as tacky and pointless as aspiring to have sex in a Wal-Mart.' In his opinion, there are few who are turned on by satisfying their lust in a minuscule cubicle amid the smell of disinfectant and human waste while compressed painfully against the plastic soap dispenser. For those who *do* aspire to the experience and membership of the club, however, you can achieve this in romantic comfort, privacy and style. Mile High Flights apparently offer three packages: 'the quickie' provides twenty minutes of airtime at £350, 'the big one' thirty-five minutes of airtime with strawberries and champagne at £580, and 'the VIP' a full sixty minutes at £840.

Personally it does not interest me much what other people choose to do on a long-haul flight, provided it does not disturb me and does not involve the pilot. Or the pilot and co-pilot together, for that matter. And should the stewardess come and ask me, as the only doctor on board, to treat some medical condition brought about by sexual excess on a plane I would require a lot more than a chilled jeroboam of Krug in return.

14

Doctored

THEY ARE A FUNNY LOT, DOCTORS, REALLY THEY ARE. THEY say the definition of an alcoholic is someone who drinks more than their doctor. And that is about right. But doctors do not only fail to practise what they preach as regards booze. They tell their patients to lose weight and slim down, yet most of them are overweight themselves. They advise people to take more exercise and avoid stress, yet work far too hard while sitting on their bums all day. They are happy to dish out pills by the bucketload, yet are rarely willing to take any themselves. And their record for depression and suicide is worse than in most other professions. You really have to question why any of us ever take advice from them at all.

Some years ago I had to make a big decision about spending more time as a media doctor and working only half-time in general practice. I had spent ten good solid years in family medicine and thoroughly enjoyed it but I was not sure I wanted to spend another thirty years in the same job, where realistically the only changes were going to be unpleasant political ones imposed from above. But I definitely craved the excitement of commentating on medical news and the constant cut and thrust of TV and radio work. General practice was a job for life, as some people said. Media work was fickle and insecure, said others. Many people tried to dissuade me.

Then one day, out of the blue, the decision was more or less made for me. I had taken my two young sons on their bikes up the road to the swimming pool, and on the return journey I had hung our wet swimming trunks and towels in a polythene bag over the handlebars of my own bike. As I was coming down a steep hill on the A30, the bag and its contents suddenly got caught between the front brakes and the wheel, stopping the bike dead. The back wheel came straight up in the air as my momentum took me flying over the handlebars and all I had time to do in that split second was to turn my head to the right so any impact was not face on. As I was stupid enough not to be wearing a helmet, the side of my face was pile-driven into the tarmac and the next thing I knew I was sitting by the kerbside with my hands cupped together in front of my face and spilling over with fresh red blood.

Luckily, a Good Samaritan driver who had seen what had happened kindly stopped to check if I was OK and then took me up to the nearest casualty for repairs. Meanwhile, my two lads raced the short distance home to raise the alarm.

Mr Hugh Ogus, consultant maxillo-facial surgeon, happened to be on duty that weekend, covering for a colleague. He was kind enough to abandon his local village fête, where he had been having a lovely time, to come and see me. Putting on a surgical glove, he inserted two fingers into the outside of my cheek and saw the tips of them emerge on the inside of my mouth. He also probed a jagged S-shape laceration between my eyebrows deep enough for all the yellow subcutaneous fat to be bulging out.

'We can't do this properly under local anaesthetic,' he said. 'Not if you ever want to do TV work again.'

And so, twenty-six expertly placed stitches under general anaesthetic later, I was sitting at home the following afternoon when the doorbell rang. It was one of my GP colleagues. Without enquiring how I was, he said, 'You're meant to be doing tomorrow night on call. If I do that for you, are you OK to do next Thursday night for me in return?'

I could not believe this. I had been working at the practice for ten years and had frequently covered the other doctors' time off for illness, with just three days off myself when I had rubella and could not risk passing it on to any pregnant mothers visiting the surgery.

'With respect, I don't feel this is a duty swap situation,' I said. 'I have had a face full of stitches. I'm concussed and look a bloody mess. When others have been off sick, I have covered for them. This time I think you guys should cover for me. It's only one night after all.'

Silence.

'Well, I suppose we could,' he said and then left.

Five minutes later the doorbell rang again. A courier had just pulled up on a powerful motorbike with a huge bouquet of flowers addressed to me. Inside the envelope the message read, 'From all of us at TV-am. Get well soon. Come back when you are ready.'

The contrast between the two approaches could not have been more dramatic, with the caring, sharing side of the medical world completely invisible. The decision about staying in full-time general practice or branching off to dabble a little more in the world of TV had been made for me. Yes, they are a funny lot, doctors, they really are.

These days I get letters and emails from doctors all the time asking me how they can break into the media. What do they need to do to get a job like mine on the TV sofa? Who do they apply to? How much would they be paid? The sheer presumption of one email took my breath away. It came from a first-year medical student, no less, who wanted to know about any openings in TV work. So this was not a doctor who had already qualified and gone on to specialize in any given discipline, but someone with three science 'A' levels and a few tutorials in biochemistry under her belt, who felt she could confidently instruct the nation in the niceties of brain surgery and diabetic self-management.

Since she was so keen, I emailed back by return. One, get qualified first within the usual five-year period, I said, if you really want to be a doctor, that is. Two, get experience. Do your hospital rotation jobs and see a few patients to find out if your clinical skills are any good. Three, write some articles and do some local radio. Four, do not imagine you will ever earn anything like enough to live on through media work alone – unless you are Jonathan Ross. Five, email me again in ten years to tell me how you are getting on.

Doctors can be funny, too, in the humorous sense and the black humour employed among us in moments of crisis or tragedy is legendary. Colin Jardine-Brown is one such legend in his own right. Before he retired as a hugely successful obstetrician and gynaecologist, he undoubtedly saved the lives of a very special set of unborn twins when one of his patients went into premature labour at twenty weeks – five months before they were due to be delivered.

The mother's cervix was dilating and the membranes

around the twins were bulging through the canal, making the surgical insertion of a Shirodkar suture to keep the cervix closed impossible. Yet without it they would be lost. It seemed a miscarriage was inevitable.

CJB came up with an extremely unusual solution, which was to use a urinary catheter. These catheters are long, flexible, hollow rubber tubes with an inflatable balloon at the tip, designed to keep the catheter in place once it is correctly positioned inside the bladder. In this instance, however, he used the inflated balloon tip to hold the membranes back inside the mother's uterus while he stitched the cervix tightly closed below it. Then he simply deflated the balloon and withdrew the catheter. The babies stayed put for another eight weeks – with the assistance of bed rest in a head-down position and plenty of uterus-relaxing medication – long enough for them to be born with every chance of surviving, which they did. In fact they are now very healthy, beautiful boy and girl twins who assure me they are studying hard for their forthcoming 'A' level exams, with beckoning careers in sports physiotherapy and law.

CJB was not just a talented and popular doctor, he was a great communicator and teacher and he possessed a fantastic sense of humour. So when I bumped into a doctor at a conference who had been a medical student when I was working for CJB as an obstetric house officer at Basingstoke District Hospital in 1992, I suddenly remembered one of his truly great one-liners. The doctor at the conference had been a particularly obsequious medical student, always fussing and fawning over the consultants, and I recalled him one day running up to CJB yet again to impress him with his enthusiasm and eagerness to please, just as the boss was finishing a chat with a group of other obstetric students about the clinical indications for performing an emergency Caesarean section.

'I've just been talking to the parents of the baby that has just been delivered in the labour ward,' said the student, 'and the father is asking how soon after childbirth is it safe for the couple to resume sexual intercourse.'

CJB paused just long enough to ensure everybody heard his answer.

'Well,' he said, 'a gentleman at least waits for the afterbirth.'

On another occasion I had a round table meeting with some of my fellow media medics, courtesy of a PR company that wanted to tell us about the attributes of a new sustained-release, long-acting, anti-inflammatory painkiller. Matt Dawson, England's Rugby World Cup-winning scrum half, gave us an entertaining pre-prandial talk first. Dr Tom Stutterford, who used to write so regularly and brilliantly for *The Times*, sat next to me. Increasingly he reminds me of my father. He's wise, experienced, witty, balanced and forever curious about new developments in the medical world. After asking about his own clinical career I was interested to hear that he once worked in a sexually transmitted disease clinic at the London Hospital in the Mile End Road.

'I used to see several of the local ladies of the night on a fairly frequent basis,' he told me with a suggestive twinkle in his eye. 'And one of them in particular.'

'Why do you remember her especially?' I enquired.

'Because once she came in for treatment and thanked me most sincerely for being so pleasant to her. And she said if I ever wanted a freebie she'd be more than happy to oblige.'

Laugh? I nearly choked on my chateaubriand. I've never had an offer like that.

I have, however, had other, less suggestive offers to join

my fellow media medics to discuss a variety of medical PR opportunities over dinner. Some are more attractive than others. I'd always be reluctant to turn down an offer to dine at Gordon Ramsay's restaurant at Claridge's, for example, and I'd never turn down an invitation to dine at the chef's table at Petrus, period. And certainly not at someone else's expense.

Jo Spink, who heads up one of the best medical PR companies I've worked with, had invited a selection of media medics to listen to a talk at Petrus on the latest treatment for gastro-oesophageal reflux disease, or GORD. (That's heartburn to you and me.) So while we sampled the special 'dégustation' menu offered by the attentive and charming Marcus Wareing, we talked about the various merits of 'H2 antagonist' medication such as ranitidine and proton pump inhibitors like omeprazole. The food was out of this world and the wine superlative, and we consumed it with gusto as we listened somewhat disingenuously to the lecture on antacids. Halfway through the proceedings my mobile phone rang and a GMTV producer asked me what I thought about a story on premenstrual syndrome that they were thinking of covering the following morning. As I chatted it through, Dr Sarah Jarvis (doctor to *The One Show* and an occasional stand-in for me at GMTV), slightly disinhibited by another glass of wine, suddenly jumped up, came over to me and shouted loudly into my phone, 'He's not a real doctor, you know!' The producer, clearly accustomed to remarks like this at my expense, carried on regardless. The other media medics at the table – Dr Rosemary Leonard, Dr John de Caestecker and Dr Trisha Macnair – fell about laughing. Very funny, I thought. But two food courses later, when the same doctors were devouring the cheese dish, it was the turn of Sarah Jarvis's phone to ring. Springing to her feet, she distanced herself a few paces away from our table and started talking very seriously and animatedly about some medical issue the rest of us could not quite make out – so it was my turn to do the haranguing. Getting up and going over to her, I said loudly into her mobile phone so that everyone else could hear, 'Come on, darling, come back to bed.' As the laughter behind us resumed, Sarah jumped into the air and started gesticulating madly, wide-eyed and pleading, holding her open palm up right in front of my face.

'Five fingers,' she said later when she rejoined the rest of the group at the table. 'Five. I was doing a live interview with Radio 5. I was trying to do a serious interview on national radio, and as far as I know, all the listeners could hear was some bloke saying come back to bed.'

'You started it,' I retorted, 'and anyway, just think what it will do for your ratings.'

At the end of the day, it was a long and very enjoyable lunch, and I would have no hesitation in recommending Marcus Wareing's fine cuisine to anybody. Especially if they had gastro-oesophageal reflux disease.

As it happens, I was sitting in another lecture about indigestion a few days later and I had never been so bored in my life. In fact, I was struggling to stay awake. I had one eye on an article in *The Times* about newly released Ministry of Defence files on UFO sightings and my mind drifted into wondering whether or not we really are alone in the universe. The MoD's files were pretty unexciting and concluded that most reports were either false alarms or misidentifications of ordinary objects and phenomena. Having said that, a spate of police officers, military personnel and pilots had been prompted to come forward and insist that their experiences of UFO sightings and extraterrestrials were real and irrefutable. This was much more entertaining than this incredibly dull lecture. I had to do something to stay awake. So I imagined myself back in 1947, working as a doctor in a small American town called Roswell, where perhaps the most famous UFO sighting of all time occurred, and I scribbled these lines:

I was working down in Roswell
As a doc in A&E
When an air crash happened just nearby
Which scared the pants off me.

Apparently some object flew
Too close behind the car
And struck it at the speed of light
Which struck me as bizarre.

To me, as Chief of ITU,
An urgent fax was sent.
It came straight from the Pentagon
Billed 'MAJOR INCIDENT'

'Expect a poorly VIP –
Survival is essential'
It said, 'Your ass is on the line'
And 'highly confidential'.

The paramedics burst in then –
We had no time to lose.
The crumpled limpid body twitched
And pumped out turquoise ooze.

DOCTORED

It wore this silver tunic
Made of heat-resistant textiles.
I scrutinized the label but
It just said 'large' and 'X files'.

I was standing in reception
When they brought the creature in.
Its head was large and bulbous
And its skin was parchment thin.

We rushed him into Resus.
Where we looked at all the data
But DC shock just blew the top
Off our defibrillator.

Around him all the nursing staff
Soon formed a madding crowd.
They caught their breath, they gasped; this guy
Was really well endowed.

They liked his purple penile pod
That snaked around his hips,
They loved his extra testicle
And all his other bits,

But as he lay there naked
Whilst I tried to make him better
I was trampled on by surgeons
Who came sprinting from Theatre.

'Stand well back,' they yelled at me,
They screamed, 'You'd better go'
But I'm a dude with attitude
I said 'No! UFO,

WHAT'S UP, DOC?

'This patient's mine. Leave well alone,'
I said aggressively,
'You don't know what I am dealing with,
It's alien to me.

'I'd like to run some complex tests
But Finance here will ban it.
It's strange, as far as I'm concerned
He's from another planet.'

The lab phoned back with blood results
In almost record time.
'What the hell you playing at?
This isn't blood, it's slime!

'There's Krypton in the urine,
Corrosives in the serum.
You sent us stools but we're no fools,
Technicians won't go near 'em.'

Oh! He was real, I tell you,
And in my heart I cheered
When Finance came to claim their fees
And he just . . . disappeared.

The phone rang then, I picked it up
And on the other end
A distant disembodied voice
Said, 'Nice one, Earthling friend.'

Well, time went fast and nine months passed –
Now all our nursing ladies
Are up in our Maternity
Having turquoise babies.

Looking up from this silliness, I saw several doctors around me fast asleep in their seats. It seems medical politics is a better hypnotic than Valium or nitrazepam, so perhaps we should have recorded this tedious lecture and played it to all our insomniac patients. Either that or my puerile poetry. The product of an immature and frivolous mind perhaps, but at least Gary Trainer would have appreciated it.

Gary is a very accomplished Kiwi osteopath and a good mate. Not only does he have a famous acting clientele on his books, including the lovely Emma Thompson, but also dancers and singers from West End stage shows. He gives my own creaking neck a little bit of a tweak every now and again as well.

As a medical discipline, osteopathy is interesting. It involves the physical manipulation of the body's musculo-skeletal system – the bones, ligaments, joints and muscles – in order to diagnose problems, alleviate pain, enhance mobility and improve general health. Based on the belief that structure governs function, the manipulative techniques are employed to influence not just the part of the skeleton and muscles being realigned and physically altered but to improve function in peripheral and distant organs as well.

Many years previously, as a GP, I had recognized that just dispensing pills and potions to kill pain rather than treat the underlying cause was a less than ideal solution to people's musculo-skeletal problems, so I myself had embarked on a training course in osteopathy under the world-renowned and gifted orthopaedic physician James Cyriax. Having learned how to free up 'stuck' joints in the neck, thoracic and lumbar spine, I then employed the techniques in my routine medical practice. They proved to be fantastically well received by my patients and, when used selectively, a

211

very effective remedy without side effects. For years my GP partners would refer their own patients to me for treatment and I was only too happy to oblige. It was a rewarding extra string to my bow and so much more appropriate than dosing patients with unnecessary pharmaceuticals.

I was understandably delighted, then, when the orthodox medical profession finally saw sense and recognized osteopathy as the first complementary treatment to be validated as scientifically sound and acceptable.

When I met Gary at GMTV's studios, we found we shared a similar approach to patients and had lots in common. It goes without saying that we will always support opposing teams when England play the All Blacks at rugby but that didn't stop me writing forewords for Gary's excellent books *The Healthy Back* and *Back Chat*.

Prior to his fiftieth birthday party, I got a phone call asking me to contribute to a secret DVD his friends were making as a tribute to him, which was to be shown to his party guests on the big day.

'Sure,' I said, 'leave it to me.'

But how I was going to compete with glowing plaudits for Gary from people as famous as Sean Fitzpatrick, former captain of the All Blacks rugby team, and Zinzan Brooke, his world-renowned No. 8, was anybody's guess.

Easy, I thought after a while. I'll just take the mickey. Isn't that what any self-respecting Kiwi would expect? So my contribution to the DVD was a voice-over while a beautiful picture of the gorgeously curvy Kelly Brook filled the screen.

'I know you have always had a bit of a thing for the very sexy Kelly Brook, Gary,' I said, 'so recently, when I interviewed her [all lies], I asked her whether in her wildest dreams she had ever thought Gary Trainer would be so successful. Do you know what she said? She said that in her *wildest* dreams, Gary Trainer didn't even figure. Happy birthday, mate.'

Even Gary thought this was funny and a week or so later he rang to thank me for the Kelly Brook contribution by way of wishful thinking, and to bring my attention to a story written by a doctor in one of the daily newspapers about the dangers of a shag. Now a shag is a fish-eating sea bird with a long neck and pointed beak that closely resembles a cormorant. It is also a casual form of penetrative sex. And therefore it isn't just the birdwatchers and twitchers who fancy a shag. Many young party-loving people today are known to be quite partial to one as well. So much so that Professor Peter Borriello, director of the Centre for Infections for the Health Protection Agency, has said, 'A casual shag is . . . part of life.'

If that is what a casual shag is, what the hell is a *serious* shag? But I digress.

Borriello went on to say that 'Increasingly a shag now stands for syphilis, herpes, anal warts and gonorrhoea, which means [pause] wear a condom.' Now we know where he is coming from. He is deeply concerned about the epidemic of sexually transmitted infections in the UK, whose numbers reached a horrible peak in 2007, increasing by 6 per cent to 397,990 new cases. While half of these cases were seen in sixteen to twenty-four-year-olds, there is now another worrying peak in the over-fifties, many of whom have come out of long-term relationships and seem to be rediscovering their sexual youth with a wanton degree of recklessness and abandon. Some are even contracting several STIs at once from casual encounters and are rapidly giving the term 'incurable romantic' a new and rather unfortunate meaning.

The only good news is the increased and widespread

availability of GUM clinics where people can be treated confidentially and anonymously, and where diagnosis and treatment is now much more speedy and accurate. The bad news is that genital herpes showed the greatest rise, of 20 per cent to 26,000 cases, which is unfortunate because, once infected, victims are prone to unpredictable recurrences for life. As the old saying goes, 'The main difference between true love and herpes is that herpes generally lasts for ever.'

15

Slanderous

ONE OF THE PROBLEMS OF LIVE TELEVISION IS THAT WHEN you broadcast to five million viewers all at once, you know that you cannot please all of the people all of the time. Sometimes you furrow a few brows, occasionally you trigger an irate phone call and rarely you come out of the studio to be met by a red-faced lawyer brandishing a writ. Amazingly, I have never yet been taken to court, and nor, I'm glad to say, has any media company had a major problem with my work. I have, however, had a few narrow escapes.

A few years ago, while doing my regular doc spots on TV-am, I was talking about toxocariasis and the dangers from dogs fouling the grass in parks and other public places when they had not been de-wormed. Toxocariasis is an infestation in humans – usually children – with the larvae of *Toxocara canis*, a small thread-like worm that lives in the intestines of dogs. A dog or puppy harbouring the worm and doing its business passes large numbers of worms through its faeces into the soil. Children who then play with the dog, or on the contaminated soil or grass, and then put their fingers in their mouths swallow some of the eggs, which then hatch in their own intestines and liberate larvae. It is disgusting, I know, but I felt the issue was too important to avoid.

The larvae of these worms then migrate through the child's liver, lungs, brain and eyes, provoking allergic reactions such as asthma. Lorraine Kelly and Mike Morris, who were the main presenters that day, were incredulous, and I went on to say that usually the only symptoms are mild fever and malaise which soon clear up. But after heavy infestation, I added, pneumonia and seizures can develop, and so can loss of vision if a larva enters the eye and then dies there. Such serious incidents of infection are rare but should nevertheless, in my view, be taken seriously and toxocariasis discussed openly, especially as rapid treatment can prevent the worst-case scenario, which is partial blindness. Mike and Lorraine remained open-mouthed. I felt particularly strongly about this last point because just a few days earlier I had seen a lovely little boy in my surgery who'd been blinded in one eye by toxocariasis. The latest research showed that about a hundred children lost their sight in one eye every year as a result of this condition. If all dog owners were responsible enough to de-worm their dogs regularly, monthly until the puppy is six months old and then frequently thereafter, a hundred children in the UK would not be blinded each year.

I put the facts across on the programme, and I thought I'd done a pretty good job. It was a strong piece but a just one. Unfortunately, the dog lobby, which is particularly powerful, did not agree. They quickly shot off a complaint to the ITC, the regulatory independent TV authority, saying it was not true that a hundred children were blinded every year by toxocariasis. They were only *partially* blinded. Well, excuse me, I thought. Does it really matter? Are they seriously upset that, because a child can still see broad hand movements against a bright background, I have unfairly criticized irresponsible dog owners? I never imagined for a moment that their complaint would be seriously entertained.

Blind people use white sticks even though they may have some remaining vision. They are *partially* blind, yet blind in every real and practical sense. Is it not bad enough that a child is *partially* blinded so that they cannot effectively see or judge distances properly? That they squint and will always have hugely restricted peripheral vision? Apparently not. The authority upheld the complaint and TV-am duly broadcast the adjudication in full a few weeks later. As the findings were read out, the text scrolled down the TV screen. It clearly said that TV-am's broadcast was misleading in that it implied that about a hundred children in the UK were blinded each year by toxocariasis. It said that in fact they were only *partially* blinded.

I could not believe it. Nor could anyone else. As far as the vast majority of people I spoke to were concerned, the dog lobby or whoever else had brought the complaint had scored a huge own-goal in raising the subject and once again bringing it to everybody's attention. At least I did not have to go to court.

About a year later, something else happened of a similar nature, and this time I thought I would almost certainly end up before the beak. I'd been asked to comment on the claims made by the manufacturers of a brand new vitamin supplement that their product had significantly improved the IQs of children taking it on a regular basis. It was the perfect sales pitch because it suggested to me that I, as a parent, would effectively be negligent in some way in not wanting to make my offspring intellectually brighter if I denied them these vitamins. It sounded like complete twaddle to me, and I said so. I had also noticed that the ads for the supplement splashed all over the tabloid newspapers coincided to the very day with the publication of the clinical trials of the product in professionally respected peer-reviewed medical journals. This was almost unheard of. The trials were carried out on a cocktail of vitamin and mineral ingredients at specific dosages, which could only be purchased over the counter as a particular brand. So it was not saying 'Extra vitamin A, B or E has beneficial effects'; the impression I got was that I should buy this brand because only *this* brand with its unique combination of ingredients was proven to work.

Unfortunately when I put forward this view, suggesting that the marketing was ethically and morally questionable, I forgot to use phrases like 'in my opinion', the word 'allegedly' and 'many doctors would think' with sufficient frequency. So perhaps I should not have been surprised to find the TV-am lawyer waiting for me as I emerged from the studio. Looking rather worried, he announced that he had already been issued with a writ from the legal team representing the vitamin company. This firm obviously had huge financial clout behind it and suing the pants off a humble GP and the breakfast TV company he represented would not be a problem.

'Don't worry about it,' I said defiantly. 'I stand by what I said.'

'I'm glad you're so confident,' said the lawyer, 'but do you realize that one of the two eminent professors you were criticizing is a Nobel Prize winner?'

'Ah,' I said. 'Maybe I should go and shoot myself now.'

As it happened, my comments were reflected in quite a lot of editorials in the daily newspapers that day, and the medical press for the rest of the week. The lawyers went into their usual metaphorical huddle and decided that, rather than spending tens of thousands of pounds on a costly court case, TV-am would allow the vitamin company to put up their own spokesperson on the next available day to express their own views on the matter, while the firm signed an agreement that they would take no further action in return. Personally, I still could not see that they had a strong case, but it was an arrangement which suited everyone, except perhaps the viewers, who were likely to be bored silly by the story by the following week anyway.

During the interview a few days later, the company spokesperson turned out not to be very well versed in TV presentation, and trotted out one dull statistic and tedious scientific explanation after another. Certainly I didn't really know what he was talking about, but it sounded like he was trying to put a positive spin on a simple commercial product. Finally, after I had sat quietly biting my tongue for five long minutes of this monotonous routine, Lorraine Kelly turned to me for the last word and asked, 'So, Dr Hilary. In view of what you've just heard, will you be giving these vitamins to your own children to boost their IQ?'

'No, I won't,' I said flatly. 'I don't like wasting my money.'

Another issue which made the TV lawyers really nervous was a product called Thigh Tone One cream. Designed to banish cellulite from women's thighs and bottoms, this brand new skin cream had just been launched and public and media interest was predictably huge. On the morning in question we were talking to Kit Miller, one of the corporate men behind the product, and the plan was that I would listen to what he had to say and then balance the pro-gramme with my own views on the cream, its ingredients and its therapeutic claims. It is always important that

219

nobody can accuse us of subliminally advertising any given product in direct transgression of Independent Television Commission regulations, and whenever we feature just one type of cosmetic or medicine we are very careful to put both sides of the argument.

The manufacturers of Thigh Tone One cream gave the impression that, by simply rubbing the stuff over their thighs, women would get rid of orange-peel fatty tissue over their upper legs, hips and buttocks. No wonder thousands of women were already clamouring to find out where they could get it. The ingredients I saw listed included nothing that I could recognize as scientifically proven to be effective in any way and there was no clever biochemical 'delivery vehicle' contained in the cream that could possibly help it penetrate the outer layers of the skin. It was also very expensive – but from previous experience in commenting on the cosmetic industry, I knew that some people paradoxically believe that the more extortionately expensive a cosmetic product is, the more effective it must be. Peculiar or what?

The pseudo-science on the packaging was typically ambiguous. Extract of seaweed is rich in iodine, which is essential for the control of metabolism. Theophylline stimulates the creation of energy from cellulite and the burning of excess fat. Caffeine turns up the body's natural thermometer and boosts the enzymatic processes leading to weight loss. Statements like these are all meaningless and unsubstantiated nonsense, of course – yet perfectly legal mumbo-jumbo for cosmetic firms to employ because, provided they make no actual medicinal claim, they can get away with it. This multi-million-pound industry is not regulated nearly as strictly as the pharmaceutical industry, which is legally obliged to prove any claims it makes in incredibly expensive and ten-year-long clinical trials. By contrast, the cosmetic industry gets away with murder.

Kit Miller, a tabloid journalist in a previous life, started the interview confidently and talked excitedly about his revolutionary product. I countered by rubbishing his claims and saying that not only was cellulite not a medical condition at all, but that the cream was no better than a moisturizer. Kit, affable and patient, hit back with assurances that his company believed they had a real winner here and that he had numerous testimonials from satisfied women singing Thigh Tone One's praises. As sales patter goes, it was exceedingly well rehearsed and smooth. Too smooth by far and I felt obliged to criticize firmly because such sales pitches effectively prey on people's gullibility. As far as I'm aware, most of these creams end up being nothing more than grease.

'Look,' I said, 'Kit may not remember this, but I have here in my pocket a letter he sent to me just over four months ago asking if I would conduct a clinical trial of Thigh Tone One to prove it works.'

Much to Kit's surprise, I then produced the letter. He seemed not to know about or remember sending it to me. In the event, because of its very nature and the dubious tactics of certain salespeople I knew, I had even gone as far as lodging a copy of the letter along with my reply with a firm of local solicitors. In response to my brandishing the letter, he replied that he had asked me to look at the cream because he had thought I would want to be involved in genuine, scientific research into a fantastic and revolutionary product that millions of women with unsightly cellulite would wish to benefit from. It was, he said, a genuine and sincere invitation and nothing more.

I was not impressed and told him so. 'You offered me £20,000 to carry out three half-day trials, which, as you should very well know, is paying ridiculous lip service to the idea of real research that would take months, if not years, to carry out properly.'

I then read out the letter in full. It said that the company responsible for the product had asked Kit to arrange a wholly independent test which they would like me to supervise. The test would be used only in-house for company area managers. I concluded that he was trying to get a high-profile doctor on-side in return for a large backhander. I also made it clear I had not accepted the invitation and never would. But Kit remained impressively unfazed, denying any alleged bribery.

'I am prepared to offer,' he drawled on, 'a hundred tubes of free Thigh Tone One cream [this must have been the sixth or seventh mention of the product's name] to the first hundred viewers phoning in requesting it, as a goodwill gesture in good faith so we can hear from them later how well it works.' Blah, blah, blah.

The interview ended with us still arguing and we continued our amicable difference of opinion later in the Green Room. Kit was not an aggressive or unpleasant guy, but he was, in my opinion, jumping on the bandwagon to exploit suggestible women with cellulite who did not need to be misled yet again. He did not even seem to mind me ambushing him with the letter.

An hour after he left the building, two of our female presenters came over to me and commented on him.

'What a jerk that guy was,' said one.

'I got the impression he was talking absolute rubbish,' said the other.

'I mean how does he get away with it?'

'None of these cellulite creams have ever worked on me.'

'There should be better regulation of these kinds of product.'

'And prosecutions too if the Trading Standards Agency had any teeth.'

Yes, yes, yes, yes and yes. You won't be surprised by what they said next.

'I think I'm going to try it anyway,' said one, 'just to see what it's like.'

'*Me too*,' said the other. 'Nothing ventured, nothing gained.'

And that is about the long and short of it. You can put a good case forward to argue that an off-white greasy substance presented as a cosmetic 'anti-cellulite' cream is effectively a con, and you can even find highly intelligent and logical women like our two female TV presenters to agree. The logical half of their brain questioned whether the cream can get rid of cellulite, but the irrational other half that hopes against hope that their cellulite could somehow magically be banished overrules it. And isn't that, in a nutshell, how most advertising works?

I thought my derogatory comments might provoke some kind of complaint. But I guess a journalist like Kit knew full well that any publicity for his product was good publicity. He was right. The TV station's duty log was swamped with requests from the public for those hundred samples. He could have given them away ten times over.

In contrast to the stress of a heated debate about 'cellulite cream', a few days later I found myself in the world's most relaxing room. That was what its creator, Professor Richard Wiseman, was telling me anyway. He should know because he is a psychologist at the University of Hertfordshire in Hatfield, and specializes in stress – with a capital S. He and a group of like-minded scientists had designed this sanctuary on the campus where students, businessmen and other members of the public could escape the chaos of the twenty-first century and come and chill out to absolute zero.

The room was bathed in soft green light to echo the living tones of nature. Overhead, a blue canopy of light reflected the calming profundity of the sky above. A soothing lullaby was softly playing in the background as the relaxing scent of lavender gently caressed the nostrils. A pity, then, that I had arrived late for a live TV broadcast in two minutes' time and I was as stressed out as hell.

According to the professor, people have never been quite so tense and anxious as they are today, and what with the credit crunch, financial and job-related uncertainty, fears of redundancy and relationship problems, the need for proper relaxation has never been greater. As I slowly calmed down and the camera went live, a sense of peace overcame me. There were five students lying on mats, their heads nestling into pillows and soft pads under their knees to promote perfect posture. They were wired up to machines recording their pulse rate, blood pressure and breathing pattern, and over the course of time this information on the volunteers would be collated and analysed in order to work out the most relaxing combination of colours, sound and aromatherapy. It would not be long before they had the perfect formula for ultimate relaxation for everyone in the comfort of their own home.

Usually on outside broadcasts there is always a sense of urgency, almost of panic. You have three minutes to introduce the piece, explain where you are and interview three guests without getting their names wrong. But today had been different. Only two minutes forty seconds to wander about the room from a lying position, describe the environment and chat with Richard Wiseman. And it was easy. I spoke slowly. Moved gracefully. Interviewed gently. Got all

224

the relevant information across, smiled at the camera at the end, and invited as many people as possible to come down and chill out themselves. Even the director said a rare 'thank you' at the end of the broadcast and a warm and satisfying feeling was enjoyed by all. What else would you expect from the most relaxing room in the world?

Still feeling serene and at peace, I returned home and switched my computer on. I saw that Caroline Daymond, consultant relations director at BMI Healthcare where I do a health screening clinic on a Monday morning, had sent me an email. The email was regarding something that a breakfast TV doctor had said about achieving inner peace and she wondered whether I was the doctor concerned. This is how it read:

A doctor on breakfast television this morning said that the way to overcome stress and achieve inner peace is to finish all the things you have started. So I looked around my house to see things I'd started and hadn't finished, and before leaving the house this morning, I finished off a bottle of Merlot, a bottle of Shhhardonay, a bodle of Baileys, a butle of vocka, a pockage of Prunglies, tha mainder of bot Prozic and Valum scriptins, the res of the chesescke an a box a choclits. Yu haf no idr who fkin gud I fel. Peas sen dis orn to dem yu fee AR in ned ov inr pece.

Hah! Very funny. This is the kind of ribbing I get all the time.

16

Radio Therapy

TWO PIECES OF ORIGINAL RESEARCH IN THE MEDICAL journals caught my eye recently. The first, from Japan, showed that loud music piped into public toilets can go a long way towards curing irritable bowel syndrome, constipation and a chronically lazy bowel syndrome known as dyskezia. This is where busy anally retentive people with Type A personalities simply 'forget to go' or choose not to go in public because of shyness. The good news is that scientists have recently discovered the 'shyness gene' that makes people overly self-conscious. Apparently, it took longer than other genes to identify because it was hiding behind the extrovert gene and being molecularly upstaged by it. The bad news is that Type A personalities – with their obsession with deadlines, their impatience and their over-riding perfectionism – are probably stuck with their behavioural tendencies for life. Many people, too embarrassed about making bodily noises to open their bowels without inhibition even in the secluded confines of a plush individual cubicle, will delay the natural process until safely back in the privacy of their own home. This is bad for them, and bad for their intestines. The Japanese scientists proved, however, that playing loud music through a PA system meant that, because they could no longer be overheard by others, a significant number were then able to obey the call of nature.

The second report, from Templeton University in Philadelphia, suggested that playing relaxing music during colonoscopies could calm patients' anxieties sufficiently to dramatically reduce the amount of sedation they required.

There is nothing new about music therapy. Psychiatrists have been using it for years to rehabilitate anxious, depressed and psychotic patients in hospital settings. Surgeons themselves are renowned for operating on patients to their favourite refrains from Vivaldi and Puccini. It concentrates the mind and liberates the logical and analytical side of the brain, thus promoting more accurate surgery. But music therapy specifically for the promotion of bowel health is new. It also begs the question whether other medical disciplines could benefit from such an approach. Trevor Le Jeune, a good mate and a brilliant cameraman, was standing with me in a hospital location recently waiting to start some filming when we heard the unmistakable tune of 'I Can See Clearly Now' by Johnny Nash playing on the hospital radio at the nurses' station. But this was in the eye department. How appropriate, we thought, and started to come up with other ideas for playlists for different hospital areas.

'What about "I Can See For Miles" by The Who?' Trev suggested.

'And next door in the hearing aid clinic, "Shout" by Lulu, or "Pump Up The Volume" by Mars?' I said in reply.

' "Silence Is Golden" by the Tremeloes? And in the continence clinic . . . ?'

227

' "Holding On" by Beverley Craven.' Good one.

' "Unbreak My Heart" by Toni Braxton in the coronary care unit and for heart transplantation "My Heart Will Go On" by Céline Dion.' Trevor had only just begun.

'What about "Running In The Family" by Level 42 for genetic counselling?' I ventured.

'Or "Shaking All Over" by Billy the Kid and the Pirates for patients with Parkinson's?'

Neither of us wanted to be outdone. Trevor's mind was racing and so was mine. We believed at this moment that there was real potential here for hospital radio to embrace this creative and novel therapeutic concept. We were aware of endless exciting possibilities. But as always happens when you are filling in time and pushing a silly idea too far, we quickly realized that there were an equal number of song titles that might be best avoided.

'What wouldn't you play on a geriatric ward?' asked Trevor.

' "Going Underground" by the Jam.'

'Hah! What wouldn't you play at the erectile dysfunction clinic?'

'Go on.'

' "You've Lost that Loving Feeling" by the Righteous Brothers.'

'Oh, I thought you were going to say "Mr Soft" by Cockney Rebel.'

Trevor was now in full flow. 'You wouldn't want to play "You'll Never Walk Alone" by Gerry and the Pacemakers in the prosthetic limb department.'

'No, nor "Love Hurts" by Jim Capaldi in the GUM clinic,' I retorted.

'Best avoid "We Don't Talk Anymore" by Cliff Richard in the stroke rehabilitation unit.'

'Or "Hang On In There Baby" by Curiosity in the special care baby unit. Anything for dementia?' I asked Trevor.

'How about Elvis Presley's "I Forgot To Remember To Forget"?'

'Or The Who's "I Can't Explain"?'

Would patients be amused or upset by such song titles, we wondered. Would claustrophobics enjoy hearing 'We Gotta Get Out Of This Place' by the Animals? Would obsessive compulsives enjoy 'Can't Get You Out Of My Head' by Kylie? Should 'Just The Two Of Us' by Will Smith ever be played to schizophrenics? And should sex addicts listen to 'How Can I Love You More' by M People? Would delusional paranoiacs enjoy 'I Can Hear The Grass Grow' by Move, or 'I Believe I Can Fly' by R. Kelly?

'Got it,' said Trevor. '"Coming Up" by Paul McCartney for bulimics.'

'OK,' I said. 'In the gender identity clinic, "Man, I Feel Like A Woman" by Shania Twain.' But now our producer was coming back with the coffees he'd offered to fetch and it was time to stop this possibly rather distasteful exchange.

Perhaps those Japanese scientists playing music in public toilets had chosen their own best songs for their endoscopy and IBS units by now anyway. Perhaps they're playing 'Both Ends Burning' by Roxy Music, and 'The Only Way Is Up' by Yazz. Or maybe it's 'Keep On Running' by the Spencer Davis Group, or 'You Keep It All In' by the Beautiful South. Trev and I had a good laugh that day and certainly kept our voices down so as not to offend or upset anybody. Trevor then asked me what I thought doctors should listen to as they write up their medical notes.

'No idea,' I said. Trev looked at me with an ironic smile.

'What about "Money Money Money" by ABBA? Especially if you work privately?'

'I've got one,' I said. 'If you're a homeopath, "Money For Nothing" by Dire Straits.'

Trevor then said, 'I've got one just for you that you can play in *your* clinic.'

'Go on.'

' "Calling Dr Jones" by Aqua.'

And that, as they say, was that. Talking of medical issues on the radio, I happen to be Radio 2 DJ Steve Wright's doctor. He won't have it any other way. I've tried to tell him I'm rubbish and could not possibly get to him quickly in an emergency but he just doesn't seem to want to listen. Ever since he invited me on to his brilliant and incredibly popular afternoon show a few years ago, I have been popping in every month or so to chat about any contemporary medical topic under the sun and it's fantastic that, among many other things, he is genuinely interested in health and well-being. In return for the occasional bit of medical advice and a rare prescription from me, he has presented me over the years with a full-size human skeleton (or 'skelington', as he would insist on saying), and a smaller, baby-size version for my desk. He often asks after their welfare.

To reciprocate, I gave him a spanking new shiny doctor's stethoscope one Christmas while live on air. His eyes lit up with delight and he wore it proudly round his neck for the remainder of the broadcast, promising to listen closely to the chest of anyone who would let him. He was on a medical voyage of discovery. I promised to test him on his interpretation of heart murmurs the next time I saw him.

Not so long ago, Steve, my favourite patient, phoned me one weekend from deepest rural Kent where his parents lived. He was suffering from a dreadful toothache. He'd tried all the usual DIY remedies but nothing was touching it and he wondered if I could help.

'Tell you what,' I said after a moment's reflection, 'if you can get the phone number of the local chemist, I can give them a call and arrange to fax over a prescription for something stronger to kill the pain. I can promise the pharmacist to put a hard copy of the prescription in the post at the same time, which will keep him happy. Usually chemists will agree to that and you can get some pain relief quickly without having to suffer until you see your dentist on Monday.'

'Great,' said Steve. 'I'll do it now.'

A few minutes later, armed with the telephone number, I called the designated pharmacist, knowing that I'd need to explain who I was and why I was doing this.

'Hello,' I said. 'I'm Dr Hilary Jones. I'm a GP in Hampshire and the doctor on GMTV.'

'Right . . .' said the pharmacist rather hesitantly.

'I'd like to arrange a prescription for Steve Wright of Radio 2.'

Pause. 'Is this a wind-up?' he asked sarcastically. I suddenly realized it sounded very much like one.

'No. Not at all. It's for real. I know it sounds unlikely. Probably a bit dodgy even. But you'll see it's genuine when the patient himself walks in. Which he will in about half an hour.'

And that's what happened. Steve got his painkillers and the pharmacist got his prescription by fax and later by post as well. In practice, it isn't meant to happen that way. Medical protocol dictates that you should always see the patient before you prescribe, and prescribing remotely by fax is rather frowned upon. But I knew Steve very well by then. I knew his teeth. So in theory I had seen him before anyway. And the whole episode gave me a great idea for a really good wind-up on whatever show replaces *Beadle's About.*

Soon afterwards I was back in the Radio 2 studio with Steve and his fellow contributors, Tim and Janey. They're always so friendly and love talking about all matters medical. There is usually something wrong with at least one of them, so we get that diagnosis and treatment over with first. Then we start on a selection of medical issues that have cropped up recently and which we think will interest Steve's listeners. Amy Winehouse was in the news again because it had been reported that she had traces of the lung disease emphysema. But at twenty-four, this seemed pretty unlikely. You have to smoke an awful lot of cigarettes to develop this irreversible damage to the air sacs in your lungs at such a young age, so privately I was wondering if the reports were a smokescreen for some other reason for her admission to hospital.

Emphysema occurs when the tiny pockets within the lungs responsible for the transfer of oxygen from inhaled air into the bloodstream become scarred and then enlarged, causing shortness of breath on exertion, mucus production, fatigue and vulnerability to chest infections. It can be caused by smoking cigarettes, for sure, but also from smoking recreational drugs, through occupational exposure to coal dust or silica and sometimes because of a genetic deficiency of a certain enzyme. It is not uncommon and leads to the loss of 30,000 lives a year, killing more people than breast, prostate and colon cancer put together. But in the Radio 2 studio we wished Amy well and hoped that she would bounce back soon enough to perform at the proposed gig to mark Nelson Mandela's ninetieth birthday at the Glastonbury Festival the following weekend.

It was also child safety week. Tim was amazed to hear

that 2,000 children are admitted to hospital after accidents every week and that six of them die. The commonest injuries are falls down stairs or from windows, burns and scalds in the kitchen and accidental poisoning. Curious children just love to pull out the bleach and other corrosives from under the kitchen sink and to experiment with all those little coloured tablets which look like Smarties hiding in Mummy or Daddy's medicine cabinet. The Child Accident Prevention Trust wanted people to make 'small changes in order to make a big difference'. That was their slogan. They were suggesting that every adult got down on their hands and knees in their house to see how things look from a child's level. From here you notice where the electric plugs are, how inviting the overhead pans of boiling water look on the hob, and just how easy it is to open the catch on an upstairs window and lean too far out.

Then we moved on to a report in a leading medical journal suggesting that drinking more tea and coffee might reduce coronary heart disease because the phenolic compounds and antioxidants they contain can increase insulin sensitivity and reduce weight gain and high blood sugars.

Another piece of research suggested that patients in hospital are not very good at talking to their doctors. They are happy to ask them straightforward and innocent questions like how long they are likely to remain in hospital and how soon after the operation they can drive again, but they are reluctant to ask the more important ones, such as have you washed your hands, doctor, how often have you performed this operation and what is your success rate?

Time to be a bit more assertive, I thought.

Then, as Steve interspersed our radio chat with pop songs I told him about my return to the Royal Free Hospital, in Hampstead, the day before. Ten years ago I had gone back there to film and been shocked at the run-down state of the place where I had worked as a final-year medical student when the building was brand spanking new. The corridors had been filthy, with blood splattered on the walls, rubbish under trolleys on which patients were lying and water and loo rolls all over the floor of the toilets. It was disgusting. Yesterday, however, the hospital had been pristine. Clean and tidy with shops and cafeterias downstairs, the building had benefited from a decorative facelift of which the Dorchester Hotel would have been proud. Better still, I was hugely impressed by their 'fifty-minute door to balloon policy' in coronary care. This means that anyone having a heart attack has their blocked coronary artery opened up with an angioplasty balloon within fifty minutes of coming out of the door of the ambulance. This makes permanent damage to their heart muscle much less likely because oxygenation is restored very quickly, and it means the patient recovers much more speedily, with fewer residual consequences such as angina and breathlessness.

Janey then asked me about the new EHIC cards for people travelling abroad and needing medical cover. These European Health Insurance Cards entitle all UK residents to the same type of medical care that anybody living in these EU countries could expect themselves at no cost whatsoever. It is a reciprocal agreement with the NHS and it covers all pre-existing conditions such as diabetes and asthma, but what it does *not* cover is the cost of repatriation should it be needed or, of course, lost luggage. So private medical travel insurance is also vital to complement the EHIC card, which Janey was surprised to hear needs to be renewed every few years just like a passport.

As we proceeded swiftly on to the next topic, Tim was pleased to learn that optimists apparently live longer than pessimists. Seven and a half years longer, in fact, according to scientists at the University of California. This is backed up by research from the Netherlands that said optimists have a 55 per cent reduced risk of premature death and that over a thirty-year period they suffer fewer disabilities and less chronic pain. Doctors at the University of Pittsburgh hypothesize that this could be due to an increased will to live, greater general sociability, reduced circulating cortisol and a more efficient immune system. The news that optimists live longer sounds good to me. As an optimist myself, I certainly hope we do.

Next, Steve let me have one of my little rants about the scandal of how much money is wasted by the NHS. It has just spent £10 million on a survey to find out what people want from their NHS. I could have told them for nothing. They do not want to book appointments electronically online in some hospital 300 miles away with a consultant they have never heard of and where their relatives are unable to visit them. What they want is an appointment within the next fortnight at the local district hospital where the consultant they know can do their operation and where their family can come and see them as they recover.

Then there is a brand new campaign to provide medical information for people speaking foreign languages. Now, while having a service to translate medical information into 160 different languages is commendable, I did suggest that £255,000 was somewhat over the top. Particularly in view of the fact that some of these languages, such as Akan, Cebuano and Cherokee, are not actually used by a single registered speaker in the UK.

Next, when I informed everyone in the Radio 2 studio about the government's plans to strip-search passengers at airports using X-ray body scanners they all became really excited. These scanners have been compared to the fictional X-ray glasses worn by superheroes that can see people naked through their clothes. Critics said that this was an infringement of human rights because the scanners could penetrate clothing, leaving nothing to the imagination, and could be used to embarrass or blackmail people as the information can be stored on computer. Breast implants and colostomy bags, for example, would show up clearly. But so would various metal objects and explosives. Personally, if I was boarding a plane, I would much rather some airport security officer saw me in the buff for a second or two than allowed a terrorist to blow me out of the sky just because I am a prude.

Finally, a rosehip extract called Litozin was being touted as the new kid on the block for arthritis. Animal research had already proved it to be very effective in arthritic Labradors, and racehorses became 1.1 second quicker over a 1km race, which apparently is the equivalent of 12 metres. Shown to be protective of cartilage and capable of reducing pain while increasing flexibility, Litozin might, it seemed, be even better than paracetamol and glucosamine with chondroitin.

Knowing that Steve loved his factoids, I now produced a few of my own about eyes. All babies are born with blue eyes. Fact. Babies' eyes change from blue to their natural colour by the age of three, by which time their eyes have produced and stored enough brown pigment to take on their natural shade of blue/green/grey/brown or hazel. Can adults' eyes change colour over time? No. That's just a trick of the light. Can reading in dim light damage your eyes? No. But it can cause eye fatigue. If you cross your eyes when the wind changes can they get stuck like that? Don't be ridiculous. Is it true that the darker your sunglasses, the better they are for your eyes? Only if they have UV protection and carry the CE mark, otherwise your pupil dilates and allows more harmful blue ultraviolet light into your eyes to damage the lens and retina. Does eating carrots really improve your eyesight? Vitamin A found in carrots is certainly important for vision and poor nutrition is implicated in diseases such as age-related macular degeneration (AMD). Does not wearing glasses make you depend on them less? No. Can smoking make you go blind? Actually, yes. Thirteen million smokers in the UK are doubling their chances of going blind from AMD, and of the 500,000 people in the UK who have been diagnosed with this 54,000 have developed it as a result of smoking.

Steve and his posse gave me the usual extravagant round of applause at the end of the interview and we said our farewells. As I was leaving I bumped into Sally Traffic, aka Sally Boazman, who does all the traffic bulletins for Jeremy Vine, Steve Wright and Chris Evans and who told me she had just been diagnosed with Type 2 diabetes. She has a beautifully warm and friendly voice, perfect for radio, and she is a very lovely lady as well. We chatted it through and filled in some of the gaps in her knowledge about the condition.

As I turned towards the exit, sitting waiting to come into the studio was Erin Pizzey, the woman famous for setting up refuges for women who had suffered physical abuse at the hands of their partners. She had come in to talk about an extraordinary legal case where a man who murdered his wife was applying to receive his share of the £2 million estate she left when she died. Incredibly, she said lawyers had told her it was not beyond the realms of possibility that he would get it. Crazy.

I love going into Radio 2 to see Steve and talking so

randomly about any number of unrelated medical issues that occur to us – some newsworthy, some sad, others just funny or cranky. As Forrest Gump would say, 'You never know what you're gonna get!'

What we actually got in the news a few days later was the story of a British surgeon working in the Congo who saved a teenager's life while relying on mobile phone text instructions from a colleague back in the UK. Dr David Nott was working twenty-four-hour shifts with the medical charity Médecins Sans Frontières in Rutshuru when the boy's arm became gangrenous, necessitating its removal to prevent septicaemia and death. Dr Nott had never performed the operation himself but he knew a man who had, someone who had mentored him some years previously, so he used his mobile to obtain the necessary guidance.

The use of sophisticated telemedicine has in fact been growing for many years. In remote areas like Shetland and in the vast reaches of the Australian outback, pictures of medical conditions and X-rays can be beamed hundreds of miles from local doctors to specialists who can interpret the results and suggest the best way forward. Simply describing the appearance of a rash or a compound fracture of the leg where the bone has snapped and perforated the skin is less than satisfactory. But seeing an actual image of it can make all the difference. For years I have been encouraging my patients to take a picture of their rash on their camera or phone, so I can see exactly what they are talking about – especially if the rash in question comes and goes and may not always be there by the time they come in to see me.

Consultants in urology often ask a male patient suspected of having Peyronie's disease to bring in a photo of their erect penis. In this condition, scar tissue that cannot stretch and expand pulls the penis over to one side in a painful angulation when it becomes erect during sexual arousal. This can make intercourse impossible. The diagnosis is difficult when the penis is flaccid so bringing in a photo taken at an opportune moment is very useful and helps to determine treatment.

Several children have had their sight saved – and sometimes their lives – when a photograph of them was sent to someone who questioned why one eye showed a bright red reflection from the pupil while the other eye did not. This was because a malignant tumour in the light-sensitive layer at the back of the eye – the retina – was acting like a mirror and reflecting back light from the red, vascular surface of the cancer. Once the redness is brought to the attention of a doctor, the diagnosis can then be made critically earlier that it would otherwise have been, facilitating more effective treatment.

Many years ago I heard about a doctor who had been watching an episode of *Poirot* from the comfort of his sofa at home. But he was startled by what he saw when a very detailed close-up was shown of David Suchet, who plays the part of Poirot. He noticed a creamy-white ring around the outside of the iris of each of his eyes – a characteristic sign of high cholesterol levels – and took the trouble to write to him and suggest he had this checked. David duly did that – and the diagnosis was apparently confirmed, enabling him to commence the treatment that would significantly reduce his future risk of a heart attack or stroke. It just goes to show, doesn't it? Spending too much time on your mobile phone and watching too much telly can be bad for your health. But sometimes, just sometimes, mobiles and television can actually save your life.

Other modern inventions and developments, on the other hand, can threaten your life. Like buying pharmaceutical medicines from unregulated sources over the internet, for example. On one occasion I agreed to be interviewed by Toyah Willcox on the subject of sleep disorders for the *Tonight with Trevor McDonald* programme. Apparently she had suffered from insomnia for years herself and it remains one of the commonest and most debilitating problems seen in general practice today. It is estimated that up to 10 per cent of all consultations with a family doctor are sleep-related and, in a recent GMTV viewer survey, one third of the population felt they never got enough sleep, one quarter experienced accidents on the road or at work as a result of it, and 27 per cent attributed problems in their relationships to the effect of prolonged sleep deprivation.

Worryingly, however, millions of people are still resorting to pill-popping to overcome the problem and hundreds of thousands of them are addicted. This was the angle the programme was most interested in. Researchers had obtained a vast array of prescription sedatives and hypnotics over the internet to show just how easy it is for members of the public to buy such powerful drugs without any medical consultation or guarantee of authenticity whatsoever.

'Look,' I said, 'most cases of insomnia will respond to simple lifestyle changes without the need for any drugs at all. Just cutting down on alcohol would be a good first step for many because alcohol dramatically interferes with normal sleeping patterns and destroys the most refreshing and invigorating part of sleep called REM, or rapid eye movement sleep. This is the bit when we dream and when sleep is at its deepest.'

'So having a nightcap is actually counter-productive,' said Toyah.

'I'm afraid so. It might get you off to sleep initially but, just like pharmaceutical hypnotics, there is a rebound effect which increases the likelihood of you waking up in the early hours and not getting back to sleep again. The quality of your sleep is reduced as well.'

'What about these tablets we've bought on the internet?'

'Well, you can't be sure what they are. Counterfeit medicines are a huge problem now and probably more profitable than illegal drug trafficking. Many of these tablets come from as far afield as India, Thailand and Panama and look exactly like the genuine tablets you would get from the chemist here. The packaging may look identical too. But this one has a different country's brand name on it. No dose is stated. There are no directions. No data sheet explaining how and when to take it and what side effects there may be. No advice about how long to take it for. You don't know if it's the real drug or pure chalk. Or chalk mixed with something toxic.'

'Isn't that dangerous? Aren't these things regulated and controlled?'

'Usually yes. Absolutely. But the usual controls and safeguards that apply to medicines dispensed by chemists registered in the UK simply don't apply to internet sales. It is crazy but they can tell you what they like and you have no comeback if you end up poisoned. And even less if you are dead.'

'We did buy some of them through an online pharmacy consultation though.'

'Of course, and you could have made up any old cock-and-bull story to justify your need for medication. It is simply a neat little pretence to make the sale of the drug appear more responsible. But it is absolutely no substitute for a proper face-to-face consultation and how many of these consultations end up with a refusal to prescribe, I wonder? Maybe that's an issue for your next programme.'

241

Toyah persisted with her questions, playing the role of devil's advocate to perfection. 'But what's so wrong with taking sleeping pills when you can't get to sleep?'

'Very occasionally, when someone is truly and deeply distressed by the exhaustion of sleep deprivation they can be useful in re-establishing a normal sleeping pattern and providing much-needed rest and relaxation. But only for a few days and preferably not every consecutive night.'

'Why?'

'It only takes a few days for tolerance to develop. That means you have to take a higher and higher dose to get the same effect. When you stop taking them, you experience rebound insomnia. Your brain is struggling to overcome the sedative effect of the drugs and becomes almost more alert than it was before. The problem has just been made worse.'

'But nurses routinely used to dish out sleeping pills to patients in hospital, didn't they?'

'Yes, and sometimes they needed to wake them up to do it! It wasn't their fault. The things had been slavishly prescribed by doctors who just wanted to ensure a quiet hospital ward at night.'

'Doctors were part of the problem, then?'

'And often still are. Although the pendulum has swung the other way now rather too far.'

'What do you mean?'

'Some doctors *never ever* prescribe sleeping pills under any circumstances because of the very addiction problem we've been talking about. In the eighties and nineties it was a huge problem. Some people became addicted after just three weeks of pill-taking. But hypnotics were never going to be a cure for underlying anxiety or constant pain that kept people awake. That should have been treated more appropriately. All that happened was that the patient

242

became addicted and suffered horrendous withdrawal symptoms such as restlessness, paranoia and palpitations.'

'So maybe they are right and maybe doctors should never prescribe sleeping pills?'

'I don't think so. Rarely, in extreme cases, a short-acting hypnotic can make a huge difference to someone tortured by lack of sleep. But a prescription should only be for maybe ten tablets. Not to be taken every night. And not available again on a repeat prescription. That is how addiction arises – aided and abetted by physicians.'

'It's the same with any medicine?'

'For sure. Medicines should always be used appropriately. They are pretty powerful things.'

It was a long but interesting interview and when I finally got home after a really taxing day I lay in bed wondering how it would come across after editing. It is always a bit of a worry that the edit can make an interview appear totally different when sentences are used out of context, and the whole thing is out of your control. Would I come over as rather opinionated? Too harsh on internet pharmacy? Was I a bit of a hypocrite in resorting to a wee dram of Glenmorangie minutes before I switched the bedside light off? The dream that followed certainly seemed to suggest it:

Scene: I was in a theatrically laid out surgery backstage in the make-up department at the Old Vic. I was the medical officer for the Royal Shakespeare Company and I was having a consultation with an out-of-work actor with depression. He looked vaguely like Stephen Fry, whose command of the English language I've always envied and who famously abandoned a West End production on the opening night due to stage fright and apparent depression.

Stephen Fry: I have of late, doctor, but wherefore I know not, lost all my mirth.

Doctor: What?

S: I've foregone all custom of exercises – and indeed it goes so heavily with my disposition that the Earth seems to me a sterile promontory.

D: Give sorrow words, Stephen. Grief that does not speak whispers the o'er-fraught heart and bids it break.

S: It's a foul and pestilent congregation of vapours, if you ask me. How dreary, stale, flat and unprofitable seem to me all the uses of this world.

D: Well, we all feel like that from time to time. You're suffering from classic endogenous depression, you know. You're full of thoughts of gloom and despondency.

S: Quite honestly, I 'gin to be a-weary of the sun and wish the estate of the world were now undone.

D: I see. Do you by chance suffer from a typical sign of clinical depression known as early morning waking?

S: As a matter of fact, the other night methought I heard a voice cry 'sleep no more'. To die – to sleep no more. And by a sleep to say we end the heartache and the thousand natural shocks that flesh is heir to . . .

D: There's the rub, isn't it?

S: Well, 'tis a consummation devoutly to be wished, I reckon.

D: You see, everyone needs their sleep. I mean, it knits up the ravelled sleeve of care for starters. It's sore labour's bath, balm of hurt minds. Not to mention chief nourisher in life's feast.

S: Without sleep I simply can't think straight. I don't know who I am any more. I'm unsure of who I want to be. Or not to be.

D: That is the question: have you ever contemplated suicide?

S: Whether 'tis nobler in the mind to suffer – or to shuffle off this mortal coil for good.

D: Have you ever gone as far as thinking how you would actually do this?

S: I might my own quietus make with a bare bodkin, I suppose.

D: You mean you'd cut yourself? Self-harm? (I pick up a 20ml syringe topped by a mean-looking intravenous needle.)

S: Is this a dagger that I see before me, the handle towards my hand?

D: Relax. I'll just take this blood sample and send it off to the lab. Should have the result tomorrow.

S: Tomorrow and tomorrow and tomorrow creeps in this petty pace from day to day to the last syllable of recorded time.

D: Screw your courage to the sticking point, old boy. We'll send the sample off to the lab and we'll have the result before the morn, in russet mantle clad, walks o'er the dew on yon high eastern hill.

(A long pause. Stephen bows head and clasps temple twixt forefinger and thumb.)

S: Canst thou not minister to a mind diseased and pluck from the memory a rooted sorrow?

D: I guess so.

S: Canst thou not raze out the written troubles of the brain?

D: I don't see why not.

S: And with some sweet oblivious antidote cleanse the stuffed bosom of that perilous stuff which weighs upon the heart?

D: I've got just the stuff. (I take a prescription pad and scribble thereon.) Eye of newt and toe of frog, wool of bat and tongue of dog. One original pack on NHS prescription. Take 5ml three times a day.

S: By mine mouth?

D: No, no, no. Just pour the leperous distilment within the porches of thine ear and you'll find that swift as quicksilver it will course through the natural gates and alleys of the body and soon knit up that ravelled sleeve of care we mentioned earlier.

S: I don't fancy that, you old quack. Throw physic to the dogs, doctor. I'll none of it.

D: Well, you'll never be fit enough for another excellent series of *QI* without it.

S: On second thoughts, give me two original packs. (I scribble on the pad.) And the usual Valium if you wouldn't mind.

D: Stand not upon the order of your going but go at once. Your ten minutes are up.

S: For this relief much thanks, 'tis bitter cold and I am sick at heart. Adieu.

EXEUNT

At this point, somewhere in the twilight of my dream the telephone on my bedside table starts ringing and disturbs my ethereal reverie. It's GMTV telling me about a breaking story for tomorrow's programme. Something to do with a hare-brained government scheme to close down a large number of local A&E units and resite them many miles away from the very people who most need them.

But I'm still half asleep. Part of me is still at the Royal Shakespeare Company and quoting from *Hamlet* and *Macbeth*.

'Can you be here for six am?' my producer asks.

'Fie on't. Ah fie!' I reply. 'Oh cursed spite that ever I was born to set it right.'

'What?' says my producer.

'I said yeah, I'll be there.'

17

The Medical News

To celebrate the sixth decade of the NHS, the Royal United Bath Hospital had recreated an old operating theatre and put various medically related artefacts circa 1948 on display in a makeshift museum. As I travelled down with GMTV to cover it for the morning programme, I was in period costume, wearing a doctor's traditional long white coat with a suitably impressive Littmann stethoscope draped around my neck. We were putting out a short 1950s Department of Health information broadcast on videotape first and then coming to me in black and white to make it appear that I'd gone back in time sixty years.

I felt more like Dr Who than Dr Jones as I stood by an uncomfortable-looking bed with a cast-iron frame on whose creaking castors patients with various diseases would have been wheeled out into the hospital grounds for the incomparably therapeutic effects of fresh air. This would have happened on a daily basis come rain or shine, sleet or snow, even though it probably killed a few patients as a result of acute pneumonia. It probably saw off a few fledgling superbugs at the same time, and it certainly provided the nursing staff with ample opportunity to properly clean the wards. Beneath the bed was a stainless steel bedpan and above it an alarming array of crude surgical instruments including a bone splitter and a very well-used set of obstetric forceps. A reusable glass hypodermic syringe and re-sterilizable brass intravenous cannula proved just how much equipment has changed in sixty years.

A child's iron lung stood in the corner, its cream-coloured steel lid firmly locked into position on top of the 1-ton electric generator below. This housed the unit that created the vacuum within the iron lung that would artificially expand the patient's chest to allow breathing when respiratory muscles were paralysed. Now, however, there were no polio victims within it, the illness having been all but eradicated with modern immunization programmes. Whichever victim of that paralysing viral illness once lived within it for months or even years would now be either dead from the original illness or, aged sixty-five or more, walking with visibly wasted leg muscles and a pronounced limp. Our first guest, Philip Whitmarsh, was a case in point. He told our viewers exactly what it had been like to suddenly collapse in his garden at home at the tender age of four and be whisked away into an isolation ward for ten months without seeing his mother for most of that time or receiving any reassurance of what his fate might be.

A second interviewee was retired consultant orthopaedic surgeon John Kirkup. He had joined the RUH in 1952 as a junior doctor and gone on to pioneer hip, knee and ankle replacement operations in the 1970s. He has continued to demonstrate his passion for his work by writing books on the history of medicine, including *A History of Amputations – Punitive, Ritual and Surgical*, and adding to his impressive

249

collection of antique surgical memorabilia. His recollection of the early days of the NHS was somewhat different to Philip's. No resources and no equipment. Doctors having to play God, deciding which patient out of a forty-two-bed ward got the re-sterilizable brass cannula through which IV fluids could be given. And, of course, which did not. A salary of £320 a year, £200 of which went back to the hospital for accommodation. One weekend off in four. Medical colleagues having to give up their work, having contracted pulmonary tuberculosis from their patients. Appalling hospital food as well. (Clearly some things never change.) Yes, he had loved his work and had happily worked overtime at nights and on weekends without pay for most of his incredible career. Those were the days. Those were the heroes.

Today, I cannot help but feel it is a little different. There are doctors who want to work nine till five despite generous pay increases and who resist their patients' polite requests to be offered extended and more convenient hours of opening. Doctors who have opted out of emergency cover – the most vocationally rewarding part of the job. Doctors who practise tick-box medicine to satisfy politicians and to maximize income without it necessarily benefiting the patient. This is the NHS sixty years on. This is how it has evolved. The technology available today is fantastic and the outcome for patients suffering from heart disease and cancer sometimes breathtaking. Yet while there is more money, there are also more managers. The whole structure is more businesslike. But I can't help feeling that holistic care has gone out of the window, sacrificed on the altar of efficiency and 100 per cent bed occupancy. It's all rather impersonal now, and a far cry from why I went into medicine in the first place. If anyone can still remember them, Drs Kildare,

Finlay and Cameron would be turning in their graves.

The visit to Bath was one of the outside broadcasts I enjoyed most because it was so different and the questions it raised were so close to my own heart. I could not help reflecting afterwards on how, when my father first started working for the NHS, breakthroughs were dramatic and came thick and fast. The discovery of penicillin and strepto-mycin. The provision of insulin for diabetics. The revolution in diagnostic equipment such as CT and MRI scanning. These days, by contrast, progress seems more piecemeal, coming in the form of gradual refinements rather than major breakthroughs. When vaccinations first began, people clamoured to inoculate their children, realizing how vital it was to protect them from the ravages of TB, polio, diphtheria and whooping cough. Today, however, because these diseases are now rare and complacency is setting in, whole sections of society are questioning the validity of immunization altogether. In fact, one of the topics I have talked about most frequently on TV over the last few years is the controversy over the vaccination of children against measles, mumps and rubella (MMR).

The public's concern over MMR stemmed from a contro-versial study published in 1998 which linked the vaccine to autism and inflammatory bowel disease. I always believed, as did the vast majority of medical authorities, that the study was flawed and that MMR was incredibly safe. Even in the original study, one of the thirteen children with autism had had the single vaccines rather than the triple vaccine known as MMR, although the publishers of the study were suggesting that parents should be using single vaccines instead. There was no real or reproducible evidence to suggest any such link and no international backing for the authors' conclusions, but the damage had been done and thousands of parents were scared into not vaccinating their children at all.

This was a mistake. Measles, for example, is not just a trivial childhood illness. It is a notifiable disease which, before vaccination began in 1968, affected more than 800,000 people a year and accounted for about a hundred deaths. Even though measles still kills a million children every year in developing countries, the immunization programme in the UK has reduced notified cases dramatically and there has been only one death in the last thirteen years. Recently, however, the Health Protection Agency had to make a public appeal for parents to ensure their children are vaccinated with *two* doses of MMR following a measles outbreak in Cheshire. Falling vaccination rates as a result of media scare stories have led to several minor outbreaks of measles infection which could easily spread to vast numbers of unvaccinated children leading to serious complications. One in twenty children will develop an ear infection and one in twenty-five, bronchitis or pneumonia. Convulsions occur in one in 200 and meningitis or encephalitis in one in 1,000. One in 5,000 children will die. Yet still some parents are hesitant to vaccinate their children. I wish I could introduce them to parents I have interviewed who are filled with remorse because their child became handicapped or died as a result of natural measles infection when they had not been vaccinated.

All the research on any hypothetical link between MMR and autism refutes such a link. There is no increased risk of autism in vaccinated children compared to unvaccinated children. There was no sudden rise in cases following the introduction of MMR. Any increase that had been noticed was recorded prior to the introduction of the vaccine. The National Autistic Society does not believe in such a link.

Measles infection itself, however, *is* a real threat. The first dose of MMR produces effective antibodies to measles in 90 per cent of cases but in 10 per cent of cases the vaccine does not 'take'. Consequently a second dose is recommended to offer more complete protection, and it is even safer than the first dose because any existing immunity prevents any replication of the virus once injected.

I have no doubt that the controversy will continue and that some parents will go on paying through the nose unnecessarily for single vaccines, which confer no greater safety and could potentially cause harm in that, because they cannot be given together, they delay the protection of children against three harmful viruses. It also means each child having six jabs instead of two. Regrettably, measles, mumps and rubella infections are regarded by many who have never seen them or suffered from them as trivial conditions which have been consigned to history. That is a dangerously complacent view.

I fear it will probably take a damaging epidemic of measles and its horrifying consequences for a small minority of children before people sit up and take notice. I hope this never happens, but unfortunately it seems increasingly likely that it will.

It never ceases to amaze me how certain scare stories almost mysteriously come and go. One day we are being told that the end of the world is nigh and the next day we are talking about the height of Posh Spice's stilettos instead. One such example was the hysteria surrounding swine flu. In the spring of 2009 an outbreak of a particular strain of influenza virus that had jumped species from pigs to humans hospitalized thousands of people in Mexico and allegedly killed hundreds of fit young people. Soon cases were being reported in countries all around the world and suddenly all the experts and virologists were threatening a global pandemic set to cause a modern equivalent of the Black Death. Tabloid newspapers talked of mass burials, twenty-four-hour cremation and overspill mortuaries. We were told 750,000 people in Britain could be wiped out. Every editor ran with the worst case scenario: the mutated virus to which nobody had any immunity; the virus that could spread between humans like the common cold and cause death from pneumonia and septicaemia within days; government stockpiles of 12 million doses of the antiviral medicine Tamiflu; internet sales to people who were already panicking going through the roof. Mine seemed to be the only voice saying, 'Hang on a minute, let's keep a sense of perspective here and look at the facts.' It was a situation I had been in not so very long before with similar scare stories about avian flu.

In 1918 a flu pandemic swept the globe killing between 50 and 100 million people, more than had died during the whole of the First World War. Suddenly, when bird flu found in a turkey farm in Suffolk was confirmed to be caused by the deadly H_5N_1 strain, a three-kilometre protection zone and a ten-kilometre surveillance zone were hastily set up and all turkeys culled as a precautionary measure. Experts clamoured to warn the population of the possible consequences of a human epidemic of bird flu and all stocks of the antiviral agent Tamiflu disappeared off pharmacists' shelves as people stockpiled what they believed was the life-saving antidote.

Personally, I could not understand all the excitement. The conditions that might promote such an epidemic had been there for the last fifty years, yet nothing had happened. The virus had not mutated as scientists said it inevitably would one day, and the hundred or so humans in the Far East who had come down with the virus had been living in very close proximity to their livestock, even to the extent of sharing their sleeping quarters and inhaling their dried droppings as a result.

This was hardly the case in the UK. In 1918, people were just recovering from a global war, were suffering from mal-nutrition and poverty and were living in substandard accommodation. Antibiotics were not available either to treat the complications of flu from which most people died. Neither were epidemiologists available to isolate areas of infection to protect the population at large. Today, circum-stances are very different. Already, however, the public were panicking. Sales of chicken and other poultry were plummeting and people were seriously concerned about going out in public.

Out of the blue, I got a call from the British Poultry Association asking if I would consider conducting some national radio interviews to reassure people and keep the story in perspective. I was delighted to accept as I thought the issue was important, and the very next day I broke my record for the most down-the-line radio interviews in one day with twenty-nine. Such was the level of media interest.

I said that bird flu was basically a nasty little virus currently wiping out huge populations of poultry, domestic fowl and wild birds in different parts of the world. I said that areas affected so far included South East Asia and Russia, although the most recent outbreaks reported in Turkey that week had brought the infection to Europe for the first time. I pointed out that to date there had only ever been just one case of human-to-human transmission and while that proved it could happen, in certain circumstances, it did at least show how rare it was.

I talked about the lack of a vaccine for bird flu and said that there was no guarantee that antiviral tablets would make a real difference in the case of an epidemic. I talked about who was most at risk, what the symptoms would be and what treatment was available. But most importantly, I talked about how to reduce the risk and stressed that an outbreak was by no means inevitable. Even poultry that might have been infected before being slaughtered could still not give you bird flu provided you cooked it thoroughly. On the whole, when radio presenters had heard all I had to say, they tended to make light of people's fears, saying that actually now would be a very good time to go and buy cheap poultry. And I couldn't have agreed more.

I thought I had done a reasonable job and that most people would have been reassured. The British Poultry Association seemed happy too. Unfortunately, that night, Sod's Law being what it is, the news broke that a dead swan had been discovered up at Cellardyke in Fife and that the H_5N_1 virus could well be responsible. Predictably, the next day, the newspapers were once again suggesting the end of the world. Just as predictably, I was asked to do another day of down-the-line radio interviews the day after. Then there was another scare story. And another day of interviews. As I was being paid a fee for each day's work on the back of every alarmist headline, I began to feel a bit like a war profiteer. But the job still had to be done.

Since then, not a single person has contracted the human version of bird flu and the story seems to have flown the coop. When did you last hear anything about bird flu? Where has this story gone? Yet nothing has changed. The virus is still out there and so are millions of birds living in cramped and less than hygienic conditions that make mutation of the virus into a deathly form for humans more

256

likely. But it seems newspaper editors soon get bored with the same old story and simply move on.

Such stories will inevitably come and go because of their capacity to put the fear of God into ordinary people. But at least it makes me suspect that all the other scare stories I read on matters I know less about, such as crime, the financial recession and nuclear war, may be equally disproportionate and unnecessarily alarmist. Perhaps I am just being complacent? By the end of June 2009, just over 3,500 people in the UK had contracted swine flu. Eminent virologist Professor John Oxford said up to 20,000 may have it and might just be showing mild symptoms. There had been just two recorded deaths in people with serious pre-existing medical conditions. It has proved to be a relatively mild disease. Yet still in the same newspapers John Oxford was ominously predicting a swine flu pandemic coming in the autumn in a new, more virulent and deadly form. Who knows? Maybe he is right. For the moment, however, I prefer to regale anyone who will listen with tales of the newly established swine flu telephone hotline, where all you get when you listen is crackling. Stories that the latest treatment consists of oinkment and that anyone not responding will be carried away in a hambulance. Feeling disgruntled. Sometimes I think people need to have a bit of a laugh in these situations. After all, we can take it a lot more seriously if and when the pandemic actually arises.

Other medical issues which I think are currently much more important struggle to be heard in the news at all. The scandal of asbestosis-related deaths. The lack of will to punish people who carry out assaults on NHS nurses. The failure to tackle the woeful shortage of organ donors.

Asbestos is a hidden killer. Anyone who has ever loved someone who suffered from the consequences of exposure to asbestos and nursed them through the last days of their terrible illness knows this only too well. Lynda Thornton, for example. She lost her beloved husband, Roger, to a type of lung cancer called mesothelioma, which in almost all cases is caused by exposure to the substance many years beforehand. Roger had been a plumber when he was young, and despite asbestos being widely used in heating and ventilation, lagging, fuse boards and other types of engineering products, nobody was really aware all those years ago of the long-term dangers.

A mixture of silicone, iron, magnesium, nickel cadmium and aluminium, asbestos has the unique and remarkable property of occurring naturally as a fibre. It possesses incredible resistance to heat, acids and alkalis, and that is why it has been so widely used. Somewhat scandalously, millions of tons of the stuff is still mined and exported to developing countries, although its importation into the UK was banned a few years ago. Exposure to asbestos occurred mainly in naval shipyards and in power stations, but its use was so widespread that low levels of exposure were common in the general population. Up to 50 per cent of people living in cities in the past used to have evidence of asbestos bodies (asbestos fibre coated in protein secretions) in their lungs at post mortem. Both white and blue asbestos can cause widespread lung destruction and lung cancer, and some of the fibres may be as long as 2cm but only a few micro-metres thick. When these fibres are breathed in as a dust, they become trapped in the lung tissue and cause lifelong mechanical damage capable of inducing cancer.

At some stage twenty to forty years previously, Roger Thornton would have been working in an environment where he unwittingly breathed in asbestos fibres. Then, just as he and Lynda were about to enjoy their long-awaited retirement, with precious time put aside to walk their dogs, Roddy and Kimberley, and to display Roger's much-prized vintage cars at classic car shows, he became increasingly breathless and disabled by chest pain. Soon after, mesothelioma was diagnosed and Roger had just a few more months to live.

'He went from being a strong, fit man who used to love cycling and enjoyed a big cooked breakfast, to one who lost so much weight and could barely eat. I literally watched him dying before my eyes,' said Lynda.

Tom King, at sixty-five, has the same condition. When he helped to launch the Health and Safety Executive's new campaign, Asbestos, the Hidden Killer, Tom spoke eloquently and movingly about his own experience. He had had one lung removed, a cavity in the other lung drained and a further procedure carried out to prevent his heart being pulled over to one side. Currently, he was reasonably well but he knew in his heart of hearts that his future was bleak. The journalists and photographers who had gathered in the meeting room to listen were riveted. When people like Lynda and Tom talk so objectively about how such a cruel disease has affected them emotionally, it always means a hundred times more than when any number of doctors like me spout cold statistics and try to garner publicity in that rather dispassionate way. Tom's son Russell, a tradesman himself, was there to give his own take on just what it was like to be faced with losing a father and continuing to work in potentially hazardous environments where far too many young electricians, carpenters and other workmen still seem oblivious to the dangers. Twenty tradesmen are dying every single week. That means 4,000 deaths each year. And among the most vulnerable workers, those figures are still rising.

The campaign we were launching was important because the HSE knew that younger tradesmen, and young apprentices in particular, seemed to think that asbestosis and its dangers were a thing of the past, something that affected their fathers and grandfathers but not them. Today they themselves would not know how to recognize it. That was why England and Arsenal's football legend Ian Wright was helping out with the campaign – to bring it home to the guys who most needed to listen that they still had to be cautious in their line of work. Ian, a plasterer himself before becoming a professional footballer, had been shocked when he was told about the scale of the problem.

'If that was footballers dying,' he was quoted as saying, 'the whole of the Premiership would be wiped out in just three months.'

That was a statistic that might make them sit up and take notice.

Ian went on, 'This campaign really touches a chord with me. I used to work on building sites and I can't believe that there are workmen today who are still putting their health in danger in later life through ignorance. The thing with asbestos is that you don't feel it immediately – it's not like dropping bricks on your feet, or getting things in your eyes. That's why the campaign is called the Hidden Killer. By the time you do feel the effects of asbestos, it's too late.'

Ian's contribution, along with those of Lynda and Tom, was sure to make a difference – big enough, I hoped, to stem the mounting tide of tragedy that was still set to continue for half a century to come. With 1.8 million tradespeople currently working in the UK, it was an important message and one I felt very pleased to be involved in.

Then there are the mindless physical attacks by members of the public on doctors and nurses who are simply going about their normal work. The latest official figures show that in 2008 nearly 56,000 NHS staff were assaulted, but fewer than one in fifty cases led to a prosecution. This makes me angry. I usually consider myself a fairly tolerant and patient kind of person and in the past I have spent years working on the medical front line in busy casualty departments, trying to calm down people who were frightened, drunk, high on drugs or just bloody obnoxious. And I was proud to work alongside like-minded colleagues who had trained for years to work as objectively and effectively as they could in what were sometimes incredibly difficult and threatening circumstances. Health care professionals know very well that certain illnesses such as alcohol intoxication and the side effects of so-called recreational drugs can make people act out of character and do things they would not ordinarily do. They also know that genuinely nice people are incredibly remorseful and contrite when they sober up enough to realize how disgustingly they have behaved. Other people are just downright rude and aggressive, and think doctors and nurses are easy and legitimate targets for abuse and assault. The latest figures also confirm that violence against staff is most often fuelled by all-night drinking.

Despite the government's pledge to introduce a 'zero tolerance' policy, in 2007 and 2008 only 992 offenders were punished by the courts, according to figures for England from the NHS Counter-fraud and Security Management Service. Clearly zero tolerance, as understood by NHS management and the government, does not mean zero tolerance. It actually means fairly generous tolerance and is merely a bland statement put out to give the impression that something is being done. There is no will to take any practical measures whatsoever to protect the people who do most to look after the health of the nation. Negligible security exists on hospital premises and none in hospital car parks and grounds. Consequently, sick children and their parents, and single women, are often scared to death in the mayhem of a casualty waiting room where drunken louts scream abuse and get away with murder.

As a doctor whose priority is the welfare of deserving patients, I feel very strongly that this cynical abuse of the NHS and its staff has to stop. Any one person who behaves badly once should perhaps be forgiven, but the hospital management should at least insist on some action, however minor, to prevent a recurrence. If someone causes chaos, destroys equipment, upsets other patients or assaults staff, they should pay for it. Why should repairing such damage be part of what the NHS provides under its charter? Surely the contract is a two-way thing? If there is a repeat of un-acceptable behaviour, why shouldn't the offender's treatment under the NHS be withdrawn? Who says they have a divine right to go on punching, kicking, swearing and generally upsetting everyone else, including genuinely sick people, just because they are full of booze or drugs? Isn't that an individual choice they make?

People who are intoxicated or using drugs need help just like anybody else, I know, but there are much more appro-priate ways of seeking that help than being thoroughly antisocial. What is wrong with a 'three strikes and you're out' policy? After that, if they can afford alcohol and drugs, why can't they pay for treatment themselves? What is wrong with protecting staff from constant insults and assaults when all they are trying to do is help people? Where are hospital security officers and police when staff need them? Nowhere. Would managers, administrators and politicians put up with this situation themselves? Like hell. It's time we got tough. I know that liberal-minded and altruistic people would say, 'But you can't just abandon such people. You don't know what they've been through, and they don't know any better.'

But I'm pretty liberal too. It's just that I'm not ready to be walked all over or to see defenceless nurses beaten up either. Thugs, louts, drunks, junkies and people who are just thoroughly nasty do not actually deserve loving care and help. They know what they are doing and many simply do not care. Surely, if they want to be part of a society which organizes itself to protect the sick, the wounded and the needy, they have to conform to some kind of acceptable norm? And if they choose not to be part of that society, they can sort out their health care independently. If we pander to their Neanderthal behaviour, we are only condoning and encouraging it. For them, punching a nurse in the face and breaking her nose is funny. It cannot be beyond the wit of man to beef up hospital security, isolate genuine casualties who need treatment and protect the staff who administer it. It has to be time to get more discriminating about who we treat and in what circumstances. The contract between doctor and patient has to be a two-way thing, not just patient-orientated. The hospital management and politicians who make the decisions need to sit up and take notice. Because otherwise, in the very near future, there simply won't be anybody left who is willing to sacrifice their own health and safety in trying to make a difference.

Ever the optimist, I do, however, cling on to the idea that one day things will change and that dedicated health care professionals will continue to want to help others no matter how difficult the environment in which they work. I will also continue to see the best in people, if I can, rather than the worst, and believe that the underlying desire in most human beings to want to help their fellow men will endure. Where would organ donation and tissue transplantation be today without this kind of mentality?

Talking about transplantation, they say that if doctors ever manage to carry out a successful brain transplant, the best one to have would undoubtedly be an Irishman's brain. Why? Because it has never been used. Now I realize that this is a cruel and racist slur on our Gaelic brothers. I realize it stereotypes and marginalizes a minority group historically discriminated against by the English and I am fully aware that many Irishmen are supremely intelligent and gifted. But it doesn't make the joke any less funny, does it? I believe the French tell the same joke about the Belgians, the Germans about the Austrians, the Arabs about the Jews, and the Swedes about the Finns. It could all be based on jealousy. As it happens, brain transplantation is not yet possible and many eminent surgeons believe it never will be, because of its complexity. However, huge strides are being made in organ transplant surgery every single day.

In November 2008, for example, a 'medical miracle' was heralded when a thirty-year-old Spanish mother of two became the first patient to receive an organ grown to order in a laboratory using her own cells. Experts commented that this ushered in a new era in which worn-out body parts could be replaced by customized substitutes. Claudia Castillo, from Barcelona, had previously suffered from TB which had left her extremely breathless, with a collapsed windpipe and lung. Normally, a donor organ – in this case, a windpipe, or trachea – would be transplanted into the recipient, who would then need to take powerful immuno-suppressant drugs for the rest of their life to prevent tissue rejection. In Claudia's case, for the first time, the transplant organ was 'bio-engineered'. A donor trachea was obtained to provide the cartilaginous mechanical framework and an enzymatic detergent used to strip it of any living cells with the potential to provoke an immune response.

Next, doctors took stem cells from Claudia's bone marrow (which are cells uniquely capable of developing into any type of organ cell) and cells from the inside of her nose and grew them in a laboratory into cartilage and epithelial cells. A bioreactor was then used to seed these developed cells in and around the trachea, creating new cartilage and the inner lining. The windpipe was then finally cut to shape and transplanted into the patient without the need for her to take anti-rejection medicines.

Four months after the procedure, Claudia was able to climb two flights of stairs, go dancing and look after her children – things she had been totally unable to do before the surgery.

'I feel great,' she said. 'I am honoured. This disease can be treated and people can be made well.'

Understandably, surgeons in all the medical specialities were very excited.

'This is just the beginning,' said Professor Martin Birchall, ear, nose and throat surgeon from the University of Bristol. 'I think it will completely transform the way we think about surgery. In twenty years' time the commonest operations will be regenerative procedures to replace organs and tissues damaged by disease with autologous [self-grown] tissues and organs from the laboratory. We are now on the verge of a new age in surgical care.' The professor went on to suggest that the technique could initially be extended to growing other hollow organs such as the bladder, bowel or reproductive organs, and then later perhaps to solid organs including the kidneys, heart and liver.

The news is particularly timely and pertinent because it brings surgery one step closer to the ultimate aim of being able to replace diseased organs with a functioning substitute that will not be rejected by the body, and at a time when demand for transplant surgery is rising as life expectancy grows.

Currently, in the UK, 1,000 patients die each year while waiting for a transplant due to the lack of donors. Recently, the Prime Minister, Gordon Brown, again promised to review the law on organ donations and consider substituting the 'opt-in' system for an 'opt-out' system. In other words, every UK citizen would be assumed to have given 'presumed consent' for their organs to be donated in the event of their death, unless they had specifically opted out of the scheme for religious, personal or other reasons. I believe this change cannot come soon enough. Having seen hundreds of children and adults with kidney failure or heart and lung damage from cystic fibrosis desperately hoping to stay alive long enough to reach the top of the waiting list, yet knowing they may die in the meantime, I am convinced this has to happen.

Two thirds of our population support a system of presumed consent and would be more than happy, in the event of their untimely and unexpected death, to make some sense of it by donating their organs to someone else in order to save a life. The trouble is people are busy and distracted most of the time and never get around to joining the organ donation register and telling their relatives about their wishes.

I *have* joined the register myself and always carry a donor card just in case. I've spent a large part of my life exercising regularly and keeping my heart, eyes and kidneys in good nick and it seems a shame to let those organs go to waste if

I should not need them any more. They would only go up in smoke at the crematorium otherwise and that seems like madness if somebody else can enjoy a better life through using them. For some people, this scientifically detached and unemotional discussion about body parts is too much to contemplate. For me, it just comes down to a desire to help my fellow man. I see it as a chance to offer a wonderfully altruistic gift to another human being which costs nothing and does nothing but good.

The alternative to presumed consent is to redouble our efforts to make the current system work more efficiently. That would mean spending an estimated £4.5 million on a media campaign to raise 'awareness' and recruit new donors. It would mean appointing organ donation 'champions' in each NHS Trust, sixty-three new donor transplant co-ordinators, and setting up a UK-wide network of organ retrieval teams to make sure organs reach needy recipients more speedily. The hope would be to raise donation rates from 800 a year to 1,400 a year by 2013 to match the best rates in Europe. But unfortunately it is just *hope*. In the UK we need to be bolder. We need to stop hoping that people will sign up and simply accept that they are too lazy to do that. Most people are happy to become donors so why do we not just *presume* that they are willing? Presumed consent – good enough. I am sure I speak for many in hoping we can just get on with it and stop wasting more time.

Yet the Prime Minister's pledge to bring in new laws on 'presumed consent' has already created a storm of protest. No matter that the vast majority of Britons are in favour. No matter that in eight of the ten countries with the highest rates of transplantation they have systems of presumed consent. No matter that just across the Bay of

Biscay in Spain the donation rate is three times that of the UK.

Religious groups, including Christians, Jews, Muslims and Hindus, together with other minority groups, have apparently prevailed over the wishes of everybody else. But why? They are perfectly entitled to their own strongly held beliefs and convictions but, under the proposed changes in the law, they could simply opt out. Isn't that what opting out means? The few who do not want to donate their organs do not have to, so that those who do can get on with it and save some lives. How difficult do we have to make it for ourselves?

There are so many medical news stories that most days I get a telephone call exploring at least one or two of them for potential public debate. But I have always found it amusing that occasionally, however interesting the subject, the story itself becomes hijacked by some bizarre and totally un-related goings-on during the broadcast.

Recently I was driving up to the studio at 5am when I had a puncture on the M3 motorway. Unfortunately, it was pitch black and pouring with rain. I pulled up under a bridge for shelter but the spray from passing lorries was torrential and the distance between the hard shoulder and the road itself was about three feet. I realized I should get out of the car and find refuge away from the busy road but I was meant to be chairing a session at the National Obesity Forum Conference later that afternoon and I would have got soaked. Stupid reason for not putting my safety first, I know.

Instead, being the precious wimp that I felt that morning, I called the RAC to request assistance, only to be told that it might be forty-five minutes before their man arrived. I then called GMTV to tell them that I could not make it for my proposed slot at 6.15am, but they soon called back to ask if we could do the interview over the phone. They suggested that they put up a picture of me on the screen explaining where I was and that I would answer John Stapleton's questions from my car. Excellent plan.

The RAC man arrived five minutes before I got GMTV's call and I did the interview as the car was being jacked up and the wheel changed. Lorries were flying by and the rain was falling more heavily than ever. Under the circumstances, I thought I did a fair enough job of talking about Sudden Infant Death Syndrome and new research suggesting that switching on a fan in a baby's bedroom could reduce the mortality rate by 72 per cent as a result of cutting the build-up of carbon dioxide around a baby's mouth. John also asked me about another medical study heralding a new test for Down's syndrome that was less invasive than amnio-centesis, and which is carried out on DNA fragments in a mother's blood. It suggested that such testing could prevent 400 healthy babies being terminated by mistake annually, as the new test was much more accurate than those which already existed. It was difficult to concentrate in my car in the rain but I hoped that what I was saying made reasonable sense. Later in the day, I found out.

Several people commented that they had watched GMTV that morning and all of them said it was interesting that I had conducted the interview over a mobile while my puncture was being sorted. Unfortunately, all of them could remember the interview but none of them could recall any-thing about the content itself. It was the puncture that was different and newsworthy; in comparison, nobody was interested in the medical research.

18

Empathy

EMPATHY IS SUCH A POWERFUL EMOTION. THE ABILITY TO understand and share another person's feelings, to put yourself in their shoes and to deeply contemplate what emotional or physical trauma they may be experiencing is enormously valuable. For me, it is possibly the most vital attribute in being a good doctor. What is the point of knowledge and expertise without caring? In my most memorable TV interviews, the element of empathy has always played a huge part and it has been a privilege to talk to so many different people who have bravely endured and lived with so much medical tragedy.

Accompanying twenty small children with life-limiting illnesses to Lapland to meet Santa at Christmas time with the wonderful charity Northern Lights was incredibly moving. The look on their vulnerable wide-eyed innocent faces as they were pulled along on their sleds by huskies and driven across the frozen wastes in snowmobiles was unforgettable. It had been the first time many of them were well enough to make such a journey without the constant attention of their worried parents, and the first time for all of them that they could let their hair down, enjoy being children and take a few normal risks. And one magical night, as they emerged from Santa's house, clutching their presents, out came the spectacular northern lights – the beautiful aurora borealis – right on cue. It was one of the most tear-jerking TV experiences I have ever known.

Sitting next to victims of meningitis as they talk so eloquently about the loss of their limbs in order to raise awareness of the condition always makes me terribly emotional. So does a public appeal for more organ donors from a family whose beautiful child will die unless they have a heart-lung transplant very soon. So do the letters and emails I receive from viewers, each with their own harrowing and heartbreaking story to tell.

These kinds of messages come through all the time and they never cease to remind me of how lucky most of us are, as we bitterly complain about all the trivial little problems which in reality are no more than irritations. These messages remind me of why I became a doctor in the first place. They make me feel humble and they keep me grounded in the surreal world of the media.

Perhaps the most emotional programme I was ever involved in making included an interview with an amazing and inspiring thirteen-year-old boy called Yibi. Yibi had been born HIV positive and had been taken into the House of Resurrection's Aids Haven in the diocese of Port Elizabeth in South Africa after his mother had abandoned him. When we interviewed him he had become, at thirteen, the oldest surviving HIV baby in the world, exceeding the lifespan of another, more widely known boy called Nkos Johnson who died at the age of twelve.

Joan Matthews, wife of David Matthews, who was

chaplain of the Seaman's Mission in Richards Bay, worked in this orphanage and soon found herself spending more time with Yibi than with some of the other children simply because he was a lot older and comparatively isolated. Joan and David used to take him home with them for weekends, and such was the love they all felt for each other that the Matthewses went on to adopt him. Eventually they brought Yibi over to England with them so that he could enjoy a better quality of life and have access to powerful anti-retroviral Aids drugs.

Michelle Porter, my producer, had been given a grant from the Commonwealth Broadcasting Association to research positive health stories in the affiliated nations and she had decided to look at South Africa's alternative ways of treating common conditions in the third world. The sutherlandia plant was one such example. *Sutherlandia frutescens* has been used in South Africa to treat rheumatism, influenza and liver and stomach conditions and has gained a reputation as a tonic for Aids/HIV sufferers, in whom its use is thought to delay progression of the disease. The South African government cannot afford anti-retroviral drugs whereas the sutherlandia plant is widely available and cheap.

GMTV had jumped at the chance to commit Michelle's research to film, so we travelled down to Johannesburg and then on to Lesotho, Durban and Richards Bay near Empagani. Just north of Lesotho, we joined the Phelophepa Health Train. This was a train twenty carriages long, each converted into a specialist medical department, pulled by an old and rusty engine running on rickety tracks overgrown with grasses and weeds between widely scattered groups of impoverished and isolated villages. We spoke to the very knowledgeable and efficient Dr Zingo and her nursing team, and filmed the vital work they were doing in basic dentistry and optometry as well as the usual preventative and therapeutic work in TB, HIV and Aids. South Africa has the highest number of people in the world affected by HIV, and the educational preventative role as well as the treatment for those already affected is considerable. Everyone involved in the Phelophepa Health Train was clearly doing a fantastic job, particularly in view of the meagre resources available.

Next we travelled south and teamed up with the Lesotho flying doctor service, who were carrying out remarkable work as well. We climbed aboard an ageing but functional single-engined Cessna light aircraft and flew further south, over an incredible range of mountains rising needle-like from the tree-covered valleys and resembling a thick green tapestry from which the black pins of a fakir's bed pointed upwards. We were transporting an elderly lady back home from the hospital where she had been treated for an acute exacerbation of her pulmonary TB. She was going back to her family. All of a sudden the note of the engine changed, the Cessna dipped its wing, banked to starboard and began to descend. But to where? It seemed impossible that we could land amid this compact sea of giant rocky stalagmites. Then there it was: a single flat-topped stalagmite looking every bit as if the top third had been chopped off with a machete. We could see a makeshift airstrip running across the surface of it, but it could not have been more than 200 yards long and there were sheer drops on either side.

In the event, our pilot made easy work of the landing and we were met by four people on horseback, who somehow managed to transport our passenger and various bits of medical equipment along a rough track up to the tiny clinic about a mile away. The nurse inside was busy giving vaccinations to a number of small babies and infants who had been carried there by their mothers from as far as ten or twelve miles away. She doled out medicines for TB and a variety of tablets for ailments ranging from infections and soft tissue injuries right through to parasitic infections and malnutrition. The work being done there was incredible, not least because the clinic was frequently broken into by looters looking for drugs and even small amounts of money kept in the hospital safe.

After a few hours of looking around, the pilot suddenly suggested we should go. He didn't like the look of the gathering storm clouds and I have to admit that neither did I. Michelle, however, was completely absorbed in her filming. I had to almost physically drag her away half an hour later to get her back to the plane. As far as I'm concerned, if an experienced pilot is getting jumpy, the time to panic has already passed. As we took off and the steep sides of the mountain fell away beneath us, we could clearly see thick storm clouds to port and starboard with lightning forking downwards on both sides. Rain started to splatter against the windscreen and small drips began to fall on to my lap.

'If I fly between the lightning we should be fine,' said the pilot blithely. But I wasn't so sure.

'And I'll have to put a bit more silicone on that windscreen too, by the look of it,' he continued, smiling.

In fact, it was a surprisingly smooth and trouble-free ride. Our South African cameraman, Frank, was busy filming it all in the back and Michelle was calmly making notes on the footage we had obtained that day. It was another highly rewarding, inspirational and exhilarating trip with the flying doctor service – a service that takes its unconditional mercy, love and care to what is effectively the biggest waiting room in the world.

A few days later, I met Yibi. This beautiful, articulate, talented boy emerged from his room with a broad grin stretching from ear to ear. He joked, he laughed and he giggled and he lit us all up with his never-say-die attitude, despite his lowered immunity, which frequently exposed him to chest and other infections and left him with a permanent all-pervasive fatigue. The love he was surrounded by clearly made a huge difference and Yibi, without a doubt, was still living his life to the full and very happy. He genuinely thrashed me at pool – at which he was extremely good – and then went on to beat me at darts as well. In the interview we did straight afterwards, he talked eloquently and knowledgeably about his HIV/Aids diagnosis and his prognosis of limited life expectancy. He did it without fear, bitterness or resentment. At the same time he spoke of his immense enjoyment of life, of his appreciation of all the affection and support that surrounded him. It was very, very hard for me to hold back tears and not to give Yibi a huge hug as I listened.

'I just have to live with it,' he said, 'enjoy my life while I still can instead of panicking, because that's what people do when they have HIV/Aids. They panic, and we all know we're going to die one day.'

I was mesmerized by what I was hearing, and when our programme was aired a week or two later back in Britain the response we received was phenomenal. People had been incredibly moved by the wise and level words of this lovely and innocent victim of Aids, and Michelle and I kept in touch with Yibi and his new family when he came over to live with them in their parish in Norfolk. Sadly, after several long stays in St Mary's Hospital in Paddington where he received many courses of powerful antiviral drugs, he died in 2006 aged sixteen. It was a terrible loss and one that I still feel. Even though as a doctor I have had to see lots of lovely people die, I cannot imagine what David and Jean must have gone through, and must still be going through, although I have no doubt whatsoever that their faith sustains them. Funnily enough, I spoke to David recently to ask permission to use a photo of Yibi and me in this book. He asked me if I knew that Yibi himself had written a book before he died, called *The Boy Who Never Gave Up*. I did not know, I told him, and asked if I could get hold of a copy.

'Of course,' he said, 'and you'll see there's a photo of you and Yibi in it which he very much wanted to have put in there.'

I guess sometimes certain things are just meant to be.

Yibi's story was truly exceptional and it was a rare privilege to have met and got to know him. But medical and social situations which I came across in the UK could move me emotionally too. Up in the Clifton area of Nottingham one winter morning, I was sitting in the front room of Dinah Lane, aged eighty-six, chatting through her concerns about keeping warm that December and whether she would be able to afford the horrendous fuel bill. In fact, Dinah, despite her age, was sharp as a pin, warm as toast with her newly installed central heating boiler fully operative, and appropriately dressed in lots of thin layers of clothing with plenty of hot soup and milky drinks on hand to keep her going. But we had heard just that morning that 4.5 million elderly people in the UK would be heating only one room of their house during the winter to cut their fuel bill, and that many would be sleeping in that room as well. Energy costs had risen 30 per cent already that year and pensioners were feeling the pinch more than ever. A spokesman for one charity for the elderly had said, 'It is a scandal that in a civilized society we're behaving in this way.'

So Dinah and I did our little interview on morning television, which she thoroughly enjoyed even at 6.15am, and she proved confident, word-perfect and extremely informative. She even got out of her chair at the end and performed her 'winter warmer wiggle', a hip-gyrating dance designed to create internal heat through muscular exercise and activity. As she boldly cast aside the stick which she usually used for balance, her broad smile and flailing arms were a pleasure to behold and ended the interview on a high note. The Help the Aged/British Gas leaflet on staying warm that winter was duly flagged up on screen and the whole broadcast brought a warm feeling to even the coldest of hearts. Dinah had been brilliant.

The next day we visited sixty-six-year-old Jennifer Ashley, in her house near Market Rasen, who was also struggling to keep warm but for different reasons. After her husband's recent death, she was left with debts and was finding it seriously hard to make ends meet. She lived in a nice house, it was true, but she was asset-rich and cash-poor because all her money was tied up in the bricks and mortar. In the current market she had been unable to sell the house and only her Aga and the small wood-burning stove in the living room were keeping her warm. We also interviewed Will, a benefits adviser from Help the Aged, who had succeeded in helping Jennifer claim up to £4,000 in attendance allowance, winter fuel payments and other benefits. That meant she would be able to stay in the house without freezing to death for the foreseeable future. Jennifer was understandably over the moon, while Will amazed us all by revealing that an astonishing £5 billion sitting in government coffers still goes unclaimed every year because no one understands how to obtain or fill in the forms.

It is hardly surprising, I suppose, that a lot of elderly

people worry about revealing all their financial details and personal circumstances to complete strangers, especially over the phone. Also, there are many who are simply too proud to contemplate asking for what they regard as 'hand-outs'. I was horrified to hear that even us GPs were letting our elderly patients down by not taking the trouble to fill in the forms or visit them at home to see just how dire their current circumstances were. As a GP myself I have visited hundreds of elderly folk who live in damp, cold, draughty accommodation which should have been condemned years ago, and which younger people today would not allow their pets to live in. Many of the occupants fought during the Second World War to provide peace and prosperity for future generations, yet here they are, neglected and shivering through the winter because contemporary society apparently cares so little.

But why does it have to be so complicated for older people to claim their rightful benefits? Why is it left to a part-time seventy-two-year-old like Will, paid for by a charity such as Help the Aged to do a ten-hour week (but actually putting in at least twenty), to make a difference to someone like Jennifer Ashley? If society really is judged on how it treats its elderly and sick, then Britain in 2009 has little to be proud of. I've been involved in an annual GMTV strand, 'Old and Cold', for years now, and it always gets a fantastic response. If nothing else, we've helped to distribute tens of thousands of simple room thermometers which at least ensure that people can see whether the room temperature is at the minimum of 21 degrees C that it should be. This is at least warm enough to prevent them from gradually developing hypothermia.

On one occasion I was talking live on air to another charming old lady in the front room of her flat in South

London when the milkman barged in with a newspaper and a pint of semi-skimmed, totally unaware he was interrupting a live broadcast. It was nice to see a bit of spontaneous neighbourly interaction between him and the old girl, though. On another outside broadcast a few years previously, we had planned a similar live link focusing on the current winter flu epidemic and had set up an interview, again at some ridiculously early hour of the morning, with another octogenarian lady living in an isolated farmhouse somewhere near Chieveley, Berkshire. Apparently she was bed-bound with the flu when our researcher spoke to her the day before, feverish, pale and generally very vulnerable. Her GP had also assured the overnight producer that she was expectorating copious amounts of muco-purulent sputum.

'What does that mean?' the producer asked me.

'It means she's coughing up an awful lot of nasty-looking phlegm.'

'Gotcha,' he replied. 'Excellent.'

When I set off at 4.30am that morning from my own Hampshire home, snow was gently falling and there were one or two inches of the white fluffy stuff settling on the back roads. The old lady's isolated house at the top of a hill proved difficult to reach in these conditions and it had been a miracle that the satellite truck had made it up there at all. I couldn't help feeling sorry for the old dear being bothered by a TV crew when she must already have been feeling like death warmed up, but she had been keen to take part as she knew it might help others in the same situation. Besides, she had told us the day before, the inclement weather would make the ideal backdrop for the item we were producing. All the ingredients were perfect: a biting cold January morning with the wind howling around the chimney stacks, snow on the ground, sheep huddled in miserable little groups in the lee of the drystone walls and a poorly elderly flu victim coughing up her pneumonia-ridden lungs before our very eyes. It would make for great telly.

However, there was one little problem. When Dorothy opened her front door she looked immaculate. She had clearly got up an hour or two beforehand, crawled out of bed, bathed, put on her make-up, donned her twinset and pearls and taken considerable time with her hair and nails. Instead of the ghostly white, deeply lined, tremulous flu victim lying in bed with a sheen of toxic sweat on her brow, she was Chieveley's answer to Barbara Cartland. No one had told her what our programme was hoping to achieve and, like most people of her generation, still energetic and enthusiastic enough to want to get involved in something like this, she had gone to great lengths to put on a brave face, show herself at her best and demonstrate the British bulldog spirit. It was commendable, inspirational and absolutely heroic. But it completely killed our story.

Personally, I do not like bitterly cold weather. I will always remember one morning when we were broadcasting live from Burgh Island off the south coast of Devon. There, the following week, GMTV's four seriously overweight volunteers would be bullied, cajoled and encouraged by our established team of fitness experts, comprising a nutritionist, life coach, personal trainer and doctor. That was why I had been there on the Friday before the event, on a spit of land opposite the location with the dramatic backdrop of the island behind me, in the middle of January with an outside temperature of minus 4 degrees C and a wind-chill factor dropping this down to nearer minus 15 degrees. I had been preparing a few words to announce to the viewers that this was where we would start our Inch Loss campaign after the weekend and I had been sitting in the relative warmth of the satellite truck since 5.30am. Now it was 6.10am and I had taken up my position on a lonely outcrop of rock where the occasional breaking wave was spraying me with freezing seawater and the wind was howling right through my long woolly coat into the marrow of my bones. I felt cold. Very cold. In fact, despite the extra layers I had put on, I had rarely felt so cold. Then the producer informed me through my earpiece that they were coming to me five minutes later than planned because the boy band in the London TV studio were overrunning. It clearly was not practical to seek the shelter of the truck for such a short time, so I used the opportunity to rehearse my lines in my head. To keep warm I ran on the spot, whirled my arms and thumped them against my side.

'Permanent weight loss is the prime purpose of Inch Loss Island,' I said to myself. I might have been cold, but at least I was word-perfect. And as the hit time was put back a further ten minutes, I practised the lines again as more sea spray flew around me. Then, finally, I was given the countdown.

'Coming to you in five,' said the producer, and five seconds later Fiona Phillips introduced me and commented on how cold I looked.

'Hermanent weight loss is the hime hurhose of . . .'

'What?'

I tried again.

'Herm . . . Hermanent weight loss is the hime hurhose of . . .' I suddenly realized I couldn't say my 'p's. My lips were so cold I couldn't get them together firmly enough to pronounce consonants like 'p', 'b' or 'm'. I sounded ridiculous. So I had to change the words.

'I don't envy our volunteers coming here next week,' I

said. 'If they don't die of hypothermia, they'll probably be starved or exercised to death by the Inch Loss Fitness Team.' I kept it short, but it was very realistic, I was told later, because it looked as if I was about to die of exposure myself. Ever since then, on outside shoots like that one in January, I've always put on a few extra, extra layers of clothing, taken a nifedipine tablet to boost my circulation and stayed in the satellite truck until the very last moment before broadcast.

It was because of my own experience opposite Burgh Island that a few weeks later I was particularly drawn to a breaking story when a tough endurance marathon in Cumbria had to be abandoned after torrential storms. Hundreds of hardened participants had to be turned back from the flooded hillsides as authorities warned of potential deaths had the race continued. Just two months previously, two runners had died in a similarly demanding Alpine race when competitors crawled through a snowstorm on their hands and knees and wept with exhaustion during the run over Germany's highest mountain. One runner was quoted as saying, 'For the first time I experienced what happens when your body will not respond to what the head is trying to do. I never imagined that the wind could have that effect on a human body.'

The Omsk Ice Marathon, the thirteen-mile Siberian race that is apparently the coldest in the world, is routinely run in temperatures of minus 40 degrees C, which makes the risk of hypothermia, exposure and gangrene considerable should injury occur and stop you moving. Obviously, medical facilities are on site to cope with such eventualities but to the doctors involved, I dedicate the following ode:

EMPATHY

I always read the *Lancet*,
I peruse the *BMJ*,
I like to keep updated
On diseases of the day.

I tend to make a mental note
Of research that is new,
Such as Data Sheet Compendium
Page 12 line 22,

But this week something struck me
That I had not seen before,
A symptom so unheard of
That it left me wanting more.

I found it in Urology
And bizarrely just between us
It talked of jogger's nipple
And frostbite of the penis.

Apparently in Finland
Runners set out in the snow
Wearing skimpy Speedos
When it's minus 10 below.

But exercise has got a price,
Sports injuries a cost,
Especially on penises
In 10 degrees of frost.

The circulation shuts right down,
It tries to keep in heat,
The organ shrinks, it shrivels up,
The foreskin's in retreat.

WHAT'S UP, DOC?

The longer they're out jogging
The bigger risk they run
Of tissues turning black and blue
And permanently numb.

We ought to talk prevention here –
It's better than the cure –
And willy warmers can be had
To keep things warm for sure.

At every race and marathon
There'll be a Red Cross tent
Standing at the Finish line
To warm each frozen gent.

The tent itself will sport a small
External hole all lonely
And above it there will be this sign:
'KEEP OUT. MEMBERS ONLY'.

19

Celebrity Millionaire

CHRISTMAS WAS FAST APPROACHING NOW AND IT WAS A SAD day because Fiona Phillips, our female anchor on the breakfast TV show, had just announced she would be stepping down at the end of the year. After twelve years of countless painfully early mornings, she would be hanging up her Louboutins for good in return for some well-earned lie-ins. Emma Crosby, from Sky News, would be taking her place on the sofa, and we looked forward to her arrival. But Fiona's genuine warmth, humour and journalistic acumen would be sorely missed. I personally would be very sorry to see her go as she was one of the few presenters who took the trouble to greet their guests and interviewees prior to the programme and to socialize with them afterwards whenever they had the opportunity. She had trained for a little while in the past as a radiographer, so her instincts were very supportive of every medical campaign, and she once said in a glossy magazine that if she had chosen any other career it would have been my own. And I believe she meant it.

Once, I had been approached by a public relations

company who had found it impossible to locate a well-known presenter prepared to front a medical educational DVD on the subject of female incontinence. Every agent they spoke to had refused point blank as the subject of female incontinence was not something with which they wanted their client to be associated. When I asked Fiona, however, she agreed straight away. She recognized immediately that any condition affecting up to three million women in the UK was important and there should be no taboo about discussing it. Nor was she at all concerned that the issue in question was not, as some agents might think, 'sexy'. Fiona will go on to achieve great things in daytime television, without the horribly early starts and resulting exhaustion that get in the way of a normal social life and family relationships. I wish her well, and I shall miss her.

Since it was Christmas, the editor of *Fabulous* magazine had asked me to write a piece about New Year's resolutions. But understandably she did not want the tired old predictable ones such as giving up smoking and losing weight. She was asking for something a little unusual and a little more inspiring. So I gave her my top ten.

I thought everybody should watch at least one film a fortnight that made them laugh out loud. Laughing is a wonderfully powerful stress reliever, and the muscles used have been shown to raise endorphin levels in the brain, making you more content. Endorphins also boost immunity, making infections and possibly even cancer less likely. I suggested that people commit to entering some sort of competition. It could be a quiz, a dance, a race or a tennis tournament – it didn't matter what. Once people have entered and obtained sponsorship for charity, they have all the incentive they need to keep on pushing themselves. What about climbing a mountain over 500 metres high? Feel the achievement of getting to the top. Forget the rat race and breathe in that fresh unpolluted air. Take in that panoramic view. Seeing the horizon more than fifteen miles away is one of the few times the lens in your eye is truly relaxed. I also thought that sleep quality should be improved in 2009. People should stop working at least two hours before they go to bed. They should avoid watching a thriller on TV or reading a murder story and instead play relaxing music or read an inspiring book. They should write down any worries on a piece of paper, cuddle up to their partner and just mentally switch off.

I advised people to put time in their diary for themselves, then ring-fence it and keep it sacrosanct. Meditation, walking, catching up with friends and exercising can fill this time, but it really doesn't matter which you choose as long as it's something you love. Spending more time with the kids is another good resolution. If we listened to children more, played with them more and got down on their level and joined in, we would learn to be a bit of a kid again ourselves. It is true that most adults forget how to have fun and play far too quickly. Being too serious makes us age more rapidly and is depressing.

What about having a massage once a month? It needn't cost much and is a fantastic way to relieve muscle tension, anxiety, depression and stress. We should all eat more oily fish like tuna, mackerel, sardines and salmon. These are chock-full of omega-3 fish oils which improve circulation, boost brain power and concentration, and keep aching joints pain-free and flexible. Then there's voluntary work. This doesn't just benefit the recipient; people who do it find it amazingly satisfying themselves as it brings them closer to what they feel is really important in life.

Finally, what about seeing your doctor for a check-up?

Getting your blood pressure, weight, urine, cholesterol and blood sugar levels checked could reveal many undiagnosed conditions which can be treated or even reversed. What about picking up a few of those free information leaflets and reading them one a day to improve your general knowledge about health? There's nothing like New Year's resolutions to get people going. You might not need ten, but one could certainly be worth thinking about. My own New Year's resolution would be to find the definitive cure for a hangover.

You see, as a doctor, it's been a lifelong policy of mine to refuse to see a patient with a hangover unless it is worse than my own. Yet it is every medical student's professional duty to research hangover cures by making the necessary self-sacrifice of drinking to excess on a regular basis. My own endeavours in this capacity have been heroic. The wisdom and knowledge I have consequently acquired have always stood me in good stead when I advise people about hangover cures on national television every New Year's Eve.

There are four main elements to a hangover: dehydration caused by the diuretic effect of alcohol, nausea due to increased stomach acidity and irritation of the lining of the stomach, weakness and lethargy because of low levels of potassium and glucose in the blood, and tiredness as a result of disrupted sleep. Fortunately, many of these symptoms can be prevented. This can be achieved by eating a starchy meal before going out, having a soft drink between each alcoholic beverage, avoiding dark-coloured drinks such as red wine, brandy and port (which contain congeners and other additives), and downing a pint or two of water before retiring. Unfortunately, in their haste to go out and party most people forget to do this. Consequently, millions of people at this time of the year are still searching for the definitive cure for the morning after the night before, the magic ingredient that will ease that throbbing headache, stop the nausea and re-energize the body.

Sadly, other than taking amphetamine (which I do not recommend) or breathing pure oxygen through a mask from a cylinder (which is generally available only to hard-drinking anaesthetists and dentists), there is no miracle cure. The hair of the dog in the form of a Bloody Mary or a prairie oyster certainly suppresses the discomfort temporarily as the alcohol acts as an anaesthetic, but in reality this merely tops up the blood alcohol level and delays the inevitable. Some swear by a full English breakfast, some choose hot Mexican tacos and fresh orange juice, some drink strong sweetened coffee and others rely on the usual proprietary medicines such as Alka-Seltzer and Resolve. There are also many traditional folk remedies such as taking an icy shower, swinging a black cat around your head in a graveyard or lying face down in a snowdrift. But take it from me, they are not worth bothering with. I've tried all three, and none of them works. (The second one didn't do much for the cat either.)

For me, after decades of painstaking scientific experimentation, the simplest, most palatable and effective remedy comes in the form of the banana milkshake. This consists of 1 banana, half a pint of full-fat milk, 2 tablespoons of single cream, 1 tablespoon of honey, 2 Nurofen and 1 Zantac tablet. This ticks all the necessary boxes. The milk and cream neutralize stomach acid and soothe the stomach lining. The honey boosts blood sugar and complements the banana, which is rich in fructose as well as that essential energy-giving mineral potassium. Meanwhile, the Nurofen eases the headache and the Zantac prevents any further production of stomach acid for the next few hours.

The whole cocktail is also rather pleasant, and unlike the traditional grease-laden Scottish fry-up, there is a fairly good chance you will be able to keep this one down. This, for me, is the treatment of choice for the truly monumental hangover, because although the only other serious alternative does actually work, it also ultimately kills you. It is based on the principle that if you want to avoid a hangover, just keep on drinking.

Talking of drinks at Christmas, one of the nicest things about the festive season is that grateful patients sometimes show their appreciation of their doctor with a little gift. These days, we are expected to declare such gifts to the Inland Revenue and I'm sure the majority of GPs are just as transparent, honest and compliant as I am in doing this. Usually, for some strange reason, the gift comes in the form of a bottle of amber fluid. It seems a single malt whisky remains renowned as the doctor's own drug of choice.

I recall being amazed one particular Christmas when the most unlikely patient I could imagine presented me with such a gift. A forty-five-year-old tramp whose blistered and very smelly feet I'd been treating for the last few days suddenly produced a bottle of whisky from the inside pocket of his tattered overcoat. Wrapped in a white polythene bag, the Johnnie Walker label was visible on the cap, and my patient told me to enjoy it later. I tried to protest but this dear old tramp would have none of it, and made such a fuss I genuinely felt he would have been more upset if I had declined the gift. Two hours later, at the end of my surgery, I lifted the bottle from the bag to admire it. In it, at the very bottom, all that remained of the original litre was half an inch of sad-looking dregs. It looked like it might have been whisky, although I couldn't be absolutely sure. I was not offended, however. Any alcoholic vagrant giving up his last dram of spirits is making a huge sacrifice. It is like someone who is addicted to sweeties giving their last Rolo to their lover. It really means something.

My special Christmas gift last December was not, in fact, another empty bottle of whisky but an invitation to appear on *Celebrity Who Wants to Be a Millionaire?* with Andrea McLean, GMTV's weather presenter. So here I am back in the present, finally emerging from my extended reverie about my medical career and TV work, still wondering how an ordinary GP like myself could ever have come to be regarded as a 'celebrity' and apparently a household name to boot. Andrea has nominated Demelza Hospice Care for Children as the charity she wants to raise money for, and I shall be donating any winnings to the Meningitis Research Foundation, a charity of which I have been a patron for many years. They do fantastic work raising awareness of the signs and symptoms of the disease, a condition which can kill a previously healthy baby, teenager or adult within twenty-four to thirty-six hours of onset. Their counselling team are hugely supportive to relatives of people who have been touched by the disease and their literature is second to none in its clarity and extent. The TV ad campaign I was involved in on their behalf some years ago describing the Tumbler Test, whereby people can identify the septicaemic rash which sometimes accompanies meningitis, was hugely successful and the foundation have received many letters congratulating them on the fact that without such inform-ation the diagnosis would have been delayed and their child or teenager might have died.

Andrea and I are a little bit nervous, not just because you never know what kind of questions will come up but because the previous track record of our GMTV colleagues has not been all that brilliant. John Stapleton and Lorraine Kelly – with their substantial combined knowledge of news, current affairs and entertainment – won just £8,000, and Penny Smith and Andrew Castle, who are great pals usually, apparently argued with each other in the early stages and came away with just £1,000. All Andrea and I wanted to achieve was not to look too foolish. We especially did not want to stumble over a meteorological or medical question that we would be expected to be able to answer in our sleep.

Chris Tarrant was his usual brilliant self, entertaining the audience and both warming us up and teasing us at the same time. He even publicly reminded me of the time he had come to see me at home with his snoring problem. We had taken pictures of him wearing one of those ridiculous-looking continuous positive airways pressure masks, which blow air under increased pressure into the nose and mouth to force the airways open and prevent the collapse of the air passages that causes the snoring. Wearing it, he had looked remark- ably like the Elephant Man, and we had fallen about laughing, knowing there was no way in the world he was ever going to resort to the use of a CPAP mask. Having tried one myself, I could not really blame him. So we probably both still snore. Since we don't sleep together I don't suppose it matters. Instead, after a chat about the options, I had referred him to an ear, nose and throat specialist friend of mine who carried out some tests and suggested a number of possible surgical treatments. I do not know how trouble- some Chris's problem still is, but I don't think he ever risked having some quack in a green theatre gown tinkering with his soft palate or pharynx with a laser or scalpel.

But right now it was my turn to feel the heat. It was me and Andrea on the receiving end and, just as every other contestant has always said, what looks easy from the safety and comfort of your own armchair at home is a lot more harrowing under the bright lights and critical gaze of the expectant audience in those famous studios in Elstree. We negotiated the first few questions without too much of a problem.

Where are you most likely to pay a service charge?
A. In a church, B. On a tennis court, C. At a petrol station,
D. In a restaurant.

We plumped for answer D and won ourselves £500.

Which sport is most associated with Catterick, Lingfield Park and Ripon?
A. Cricket, B. Football, C. Greyhound racing, D. Horse racing.

Andrea and I had both had a little flutter on the horses before now, so it wasn't too difficult to select answer D. We were now on £1,000.

Which former Blue Peter *presenter was the mother of a famous daughter called Sophie?*
A. Valerie Singleton, B. Tina Heath, C. Janet Ellis, D. Lesley Judd.

It was not hard to come up with Janet Ellis to double our money to £2,000. The relief in getting that far was tangible. We would at least now not always be remembered as the first celebrity pair ever to fall at the first hurdle on *Millionaire* and come away with nothing. We would not be eternal laughing stocks. The next question, for £5,000, was about wine.

293

Which of these words refers to someone who cultivates grapes for winemaking?
A. Horticulturist, B. Viniculturist, C. Aquaculturist, D. Apiculturist.

With all the drinking both of us had enjoyed over the years, it would have been criminal if we had not known what a viniculturist did for a living. Now we were on a roll. Next up, for £10,000, we had a question about birds.

Which type of waterbird shares its name with a shade of blue?
A. Coot, B. Grebe, C. Mallard, D. Teal.

Andrea surprised me by describing the colours of a coot and mallard, and teal blue sounded good to both of us. Now we were on £10,000 and we had not yet used any lifelines. Next up, we had a question about RazorLight.

In 2006 RazorLight topped the charts with which song?
A. 'Canada', B. 'South Africa', C. 'Australia', D. 'America'.

Luckily, I had been reading out dedications and pledges of money on Steve Wright's show on Radio 2 for Children in Need a few weeks previously, so I was fairly sure that it was 'America'. Andrea, however, thought it was 'Australia'. I told Chris that there was a little bit of the neurosurgeon in me that did not want to do something I was not completely sure of. If a neurosurgeon does that, I explained, he kills the patient. The audience found this quite funny. So we used one of our lifelines and asked them, and 92 per cent of them agreed with me that the answer was 'America'. The audience in fact were terrific, knowledgeable on popular music and TV soaps especially and very welcoming at the start and end of the show.

Then came the £50,000 question.

Who became Scotland's first First Minister in 1999?
A. Robin Cook, B. Donald Dewar, C. David Steel, D. Tam Dalyell.

I was pretty sure I knew this. I'd stood under a fifteen-foot statue of Donald Dewar in a Glasgow shopping centre and remembered it because of an orange traffic cone that someone had climbed up the statue to put over his head. I had subsequently heard that the cone was resident in that position more often then not. As soon as the police remove it, some joker scales the statue again and replaces it. Yet I could not be 100 per cent sure of the answer and it was the two charities that would lose out if I gambled unnecessarily when we still had two lifelines left. So Andrea and I decided we would phone a friend in the shape of Peter McHugh, our boss and director of programmes at GMTV.

'Will he know this?' asked Chris.

'For sure.'

'Is he smart?'

'He employed *us*, didn't he?'

The repartee certainly helped calm the nerves a little, and we felt the audience willing us on. The phone rang. Peter picked up.

'Peter McHugh.'

Chris, who knew Peter pretty well through TV programmes in the past, then embarked on a cosy little chat with him, mainly at our expense. As soon as he heard us asking the question, he immediately knew the answer.

'Donald Dewar.'

'Thanks, Peter. And can we have a pay rise?' I asked. But the line had suddenly gone dead. Now we were up to an exciting £50,000, a figure we were delighted with as we knew it would make a significant difference to each charity. A cheque to guarantee that amount was brandished in front of us by a grinning and congratulatory Tarrant. The next question was worth £75,000.

Who won the Academy Award for Best Director in 2008?
A. Joel and Ethan Coen, B. Julian Schnabel, C. Tony Gilroy,
D. Paul Thomas Anderson.

Wow. This was a difficult one. Neither Andrea nor I had heard of the last two at all. After a little debate, we used our 50/50 lifeline and answers B and C were removed. We had heard of the Coen brothers but not of Paul Thomas Anderson, and since we were guaranteed £50,000 anyway we opted for answer A. We were over the moon when this was proved correct.

The next question, if we got it right, could elevate us to £150,000 but if we were to get it wrong it would take us back to only £50,000. We could still lose £25,000 if we were not careful and it worried us. Tarrant read the question.

Which African city lies just north of Lake Victoria?
A. Khartoum, B. Kampala, C. Kigali, D. Kinshasa.

I felt a surge of excitement run through me, which Chris immediately picked up on.

'Dr Hilary has a smug expression on his face,' he said. And he was definitely not wrong. I didn't know the answer myself but I *did* know that Andrea had lived in Kenya as a child, not very far from the shores of Lake Victoria, and I

296

was confident that she would know the answer to this one. As I glanced towards her, she looked calm, just staring straight ahead. Her face was inscrutable, neither excited nor smiling nor concerned. She was clearly weighing up some doubts in her own mind.

'I think I know, but I'm not absolutely certain,' she said. 'There's a risk we could lose £25,000.'

'But to reach £150,000 would be phenomenal. And a huge step up for the charities. How sure are you?' I asked.

'Pretty sure.'

'I think you should go with your heart. Go with your instincts. We could lose a little, I know, but gain a lot too. It sounds like a reasonable gamble.'

Luckily, once again Andrea agreed. All through the show we had deferred to each other and thought out our next moves fairly logically. We had been lucky too. So much depends on the questions. You can be an intellectual giant like Stephen Hawking and still come to grief over a £100 question on *Emmerdale*. *Millionaire* is a lottery, after all, but a very entertaining one, and a brilliant format which is now sold in hundreds of countries across the world. We announced our final answer.

'Kampala,' said Andrea.

Tarrant looked at us both enigmatically as the familiar three-tone chord signalled our response on the screen.

'If you'd said Khartoum, you'd have *lost* £25,000,' he said.

'If you'd said Kigali, you'd have just *lost* £25,000.

'You said Kampala.' The tension was now unbearable, and Chris was milking it for all it was worth. 'You were on £75,000, and you have just *lost* £75,000 . . . (long pause and sigh of disappointment from the audience) because you've *won* £150,000.'

We could not believe it. The audience were clapping loudly and we gave each other a big kiss on the cheek. Result. This was getting better by the minute. Surely we could not mess it all up now? We had secured £75,000 for each charity. But then, for £250,000, came the killer.

In Greek mythology, which of these was a giant with a hundred eyes?
A. Argus, B. Daphnis, C. Agamemnon, D. Narcissus.

Tricky. We obviously did not know. Was there a clue in the names, Andrea asked me. Anything medical? Sadly not. We had £150,000 in the bank and were not going to lose it now on a one-in-four risky guess. We were delighted with the cheque which we knew would be so constructively used by the charities, and thanked Tarrant accordingly.

'If you *had* answered, which would you have chosen?' he inevitably asked.

'I don't think it's Narcissus,' said Andrea.

'No. He just looked into the water and saw a reflection of himself which turned him to stone, didn't it?' I mused. 'And I don't think it's Agamemnon because it just doesn't ring any bells.'

'I think it's Argus,' said Andrea.

'You're only saying that because you've just received their Christmas catalogue!' joked Chris.

'Daphnis,' I said.

But, as it turned out, Andrea's guess was the right one, and on hearing the answer we said cheerio to the audience and repaired to the Green Room for a celebratory glass of wine, courtesy of some expert viniculturist from France.

Index

bacon, carcinogenic properties
104–5
Ballesteros, Severiano 92
banana milkshake, hangover cure
289–90
bariatric surgery 177–81
Barr, Roseanne 178
basal cell carcinoma 14–17
Basingstoke District Hospital 204
'Beach Surgery' 20
Beadle's About 232
Beatie, Thomas 19–22
Beckham, Victoria 42
Beechdown 174
Bell's palsy 125
benefits, unclaimed 277–8
beta-blockers 190
Bevan, Aneurin 145
Big Dave 104–5
Bikini Diet 165
binge-drinking 1, 154–60
bio-engineering 265
bipolar disorder 12
Birchall, Professor Martin 265–6
bird flu 254–7
Black Museum, Scotland Yard 50
bladder 51
Blair, Tony 137
bleeding 24–9, 60
blindness 216–17, 237
blood sugar levels 186
BMI Healthcare 225
Boazman, Sally 237
bone diseases 45, 126
Born Free Organization 5
Borriello, Professor Peter 213
Bournemouth 63–5, 173
bowel problems 39–41, 226–7
boxing 11–14, 25
Bradford football stadium fire 91
brain
haemorrhage 25–6, 60
status epilepticus 193–6

transplants 264
tumours 92–7
Bramley, Darren 128–9
breast cancer 9, 15, 45
breastfeeding, wet nurses 20–2
Breatharians 22–4
Brinton, Jessica 184
British Association of Aesthetic
Plastic Surgeons (BAAPS) 183
British Association of Cosmetic
Surgeons (BACS) 183
British Gas 277
British Journal of Sexual Medicine
184, 198
British Petroleum 194
British Poultry Association 255–6
Britton, Fern 150, 177, 179
bronchitis 74–5
Brook, Kelly 212–13
Brooke, Zinzan 212
Brown, Gordon 103–4, 137, 266, 267
Bruni, Carla 185
Bruno, Frank 11–14
Buddhism 5
bulimia 9
bunions 31
BUPA 186
bureaucracy 66–7
Burgh Island 280–2
burns 91

Caestecker, Dr John de 206
caffeine 220
California, University of 235
Cambridge University 30
Campbell, Alastair 137
Campbell, Naomi 9
cancer 179
breast 9, 15, 45
colorectal 39
head and neck 140–2
lung 52, 258–60
prostate 38–9